1989

Determinants
of
HMO
Success

Determinants of HMO Success

Peter D. Fox
LuAnn Heinen
with Richard J. Steele

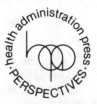

Health Administration Press Perspectives • Ann Arbor, Michigan 1987

Printed in the United States of America.

Library of Congress Cataloging-in-Publication Data

Fox, Peter D.
  Determinants of HMO success.

  1. Health maintenance organizations—United States—Administration.
2. Medical care—United States—Cost effectiveness.   3. Health
maintenance organizations—United States—Case studies.   I. Heinen,
LuAnn.   II. Steele, Richard J.   III. Title.   (DNLM: 1. Health
Maintenance Organizations—United States. W 275 AA1 F73]
RA413.5.U5F676 1987   362.1' 0425   86–29553
ISBN 0–910701–21–0 (pbk.)

Health Administration Press
Perspectives is an imprint of Health
Administration Press dedicated to
books and other material of timely
and special interest for health
care practitioners.

Health Administration Press
A Division of the Foundation of the
American College of Healthcare Executives
1021 East Huron Street
Ann Arbor, Michigan 48104-9990

Table of Contents

Part IV Lifeguard

Part V Harvard Community Health Plan

List of Tables

Preface

In recent years, enrollment in health maintenance organizations (HMOs) has grown at a rapid rate; in fact, new HMOs are being formed regularly. At the same time, many observers now predict greater competition, both among HMOs and between HMOs and other, newer systems that combine health care financing and delivery. Interestingly, the cost management techniques adopted by these new systems as well as by employers and health insurers in their standard health benefits programs were more often than not pioneered by HMOs. Thus the lessons from the most successful HMOs become increasingly important, both for other HMOs (particularly those in the early stages of development) and for various organizations engaged in cost management. However, there has been little systematic study of the best practices of successful HMOs.

Between 1983 and 1985, Lewin and Associates, Inc., and Birch & Davis Associates, Inc., under contract with the Office of Health Maintenance Organizations in the U.S. Department of Health and Human Services, studied eight successful HMOs and documented their best practices. This book contains a synthesis of our findings from the eight case studies and attempts to distill the essential qualities shared by these HMOs. It also presents four of the case studies, selected to represent a diversity of origins and organizational structures.

A number of changes have occurred since 1985. SHARE Development Corporation, the parent company of SHARE-Minnesota, has merged with United HealthCare Corporation; Maxicare

Health Plans, the parent company of Maxicare California, has acquired two other publicly held HMO firms, HealthAmerica and HealthCare USA; United States Health Care Systems, Inc., has both shortened its name to U. S. Healthcare and initiated, and subsequently terminated, an innovative joint venture with the Lincoln National Insurance Company; and several of the plans are taking the first steps to broaden their product lines beyond the pure HMO. The field is likely to remain dynamic. Nonetheless, we believe that the essential qualities we have sought to document will remain critical to success in the foreseeable future. It should also be noted that the data in this book are in most cases valid through 1984 or 1985, although some more recent information has been incorporated immediately prior to publication.

The study benefited tremendously from the support and guidance of Beth Roy, director of the Division of Qualification, Office of Health Maintenance Organizations at the time of the study. (She is currently regional vice president of eastern operations, Lincoln National Insurance Company.) Her creative insights, participation in several of the site visits, and careful reading of earlier drafts contributed enormously to this report. Above all, her vision of what the study could accomplish was a source of inspiration.

We are also indebted to the members of the study's advisory board, each of whom devoted time and energy to ensuring the accuracy and usefulness of the final product. Several of them also hosted site visits. We note the contributions of: Harris Berman, M.D., executive director, Matthew Thornton Health Plan, Inc.; Richard Cannon, executive vice president, Harvard Community Health Plan; Dorothy Emerson-O'Neill, executive vice president, Lifeguard HMO; Jack Shelton, manager, Employee Insurance Department, Ford Motor Company; Fred Wasserman, chairman, Maxicare Health Plans, Inc.; and Jeffrey Weiner, M.D., executive vice president, Medical Delivery Systems, U. S. Healthcare.

We also acknowledge the special assistance of Kenneth Linde, vice president of operations for the northern division of Travelers Health Plan. He played a key role in the development and early management of this project in his former capacity as director of the Division of Qualification in the Office of HMOs.

In addition, the Group Health Association of America performed a review of the literature as background for the study, and George Strumpf, its deputy executive director at the time, critiqued various drafts. (Strumpf is now director of government relations in the Washington office of the Health Insurance Plan of Greater New York.)

Finally, we are grateful to the eight plans that participated in the project. Each of them was host to us for several days and later reviewed drafts of both part I of this book and the case studies of their own plans. Their willingness to invest time and to be open with us made the study possible.

Any views expressed herein are those of the authors alone and do not necessarily reflect the positions or policies of the U.S. Department of Health and Human Services.

Part I
Overview

1

Introduction

Enrollment in HMOs rose at the unprecedented rate of 24.9 percent between July 1984 and June 1985, reaching 18.9 million, more than double the June 1980 enrollment of 9.1 million.[1] Enrollment growth has also exceeded 10 percent in seven of the last eight years, an enviable track record by any standard. Furthermore, the financial situation of both for-profit and nonprofit HMOs has never been healthier.

As is true in any sector of the economy, some HMOs have performed better than others, and a few have become insolvent.[2] Although HMO growth is so great that it is straining the management capacities of many plans, competition among HMOs is intensifying, suggesting the need for even sharper decision making.

In this book we attempt to identify factors that characterize successful HMOs. We offer an overview of some of the areas that are of concern to plans and that are viewed as key to their success. In addition, we describe specific management principles and practices and give examples of how these principles and practices are articulated.

Eight individual plans were studied:

— Bay Pacific Health Plan, San Bruno, California
— Capital Area Community Health Plan, Latham, New York
— Harvard Community Health Plan (HCHP), Boston, Massachusetts
— HMO of Pennsylvania (HMO-PA), Blue Bell, Pennsylvania

— Lifeguard HMO, Campbell, California

— Maxicare California, Los Angeles, California

— Rhode Island Group Health Association (RIGHA), Providence, Rhode Island

— SHARE-Minnesota, Bloomington, Minnesota

Two caveats are in order. First, our intent is primarily to understand factors leading to success as reported by HMO representatives. Although our own perspectives are reflected, we have not attempted to perform an independent assessment or audit of the organizations' performance. Our interview protocol included questions about weaknesses, problems, and mistakes, but we did not talk to enrollees, competitors, employers, or others who might inject a note of skepticism. Nonetheless, we believe that, by understanding and articulating the best practices of successful HMOs, we can assist others who might wish to follow in their footsteps.

Second, it has been suggested that the major determinant of success may be charismatic leadership or generically superior management, whose characteristics cannot readily be measured. However, leadership qualities alone, vaguely defined, do not generate success; they simply create fertile environments that facilitate it. Leaders must take concrete steps, make specific decisions, and institute observable policies and structures.

One stimulus for this effort was the widely read book, *In Search of Excellence.*[3] Midway through our study, *Business Week* had a cover story entitled "OOPS."[4] It reported that a significant number of companies cited in that book as paragons of excellence had performed poorly in the year following its publication. Robert Waterman, one of the authors, commented in a letter to the editor of *Business Week*:

> We never tried to find, nor expected to find, formulas for success. With only a couple of exceptions, we have no regrets about our choice of companies. All were well-regarded by informed observers of the business scene. All had outperformed their industry for 20 years on a variety of financial measures. But fine athletes age, industries mature and decline, and long runs on Broadway eventually end. Anyone who believes in fomulas for success, or forever excellence, is nuts.[5]

It is possible that some of the HMOs in our sample may be on next year's oops list. Nonetheless, we believe they are doing certain things right, things that others will benefit from emulating.

Notes

1. InterStudy, *National HMO Census 1982* and *The HMO Summary: June 1985* (Excelsior, Minn.: InterStudy, 1983 and 1985).

2. Since 1973, approximately 30 HMOs have ceased operations or merged with another organization for financial reasons (U.S. Public Health Service, Office of Health Maintenance Organizations, personal communication, 1986).

3. Thomas J. Peters and Robert H. Waterman, Jr., *In Search of Excellence* (New York: Warner Books, 1982).

4. "Who's Excellent Now?" *Business Week*, 5 November 1984, pp. 76–78.

5. *Business Week*, 26 November 1984, p. 9.

2

Study Design

Definition of Success and Selection of HMOs

Like beauty, success is in the eye of the beholder. We made no attempt, therefore, to impose a rigid definition of success in selecting our sample. Rather, we sought to identify plans that were considered to be outstanding among their peers and that had a record of market acceptance and excellent financial performance. With a sample of only eight HMOs, it was not possible to represent the industry as a whole nor to include all the outstanding plans, although we did strive for a broad representation of types of delivery systems, a mix of for-profits and nonprofits, and both national and local entities.

As a first step in the selection process, we decided to limit the sample to HMOs that have achieved success in the relatively recent past (15 years or less). This was because we viewed the primary audience of the study as HMO managers and board members in new plans or in plans approaching critical growth stages. The HMOs that were excluded were formed in a very different environment and therefore were not necessarily representative of the characteristics that lead to success in today's more competitive marketplace. Also excluded were HMOs with fewer than 25,000 members as of January 1984, as well as those that had been operational for less than five years, because we wanted to study mature plans and observe how they grew, overcame obstacles, and stayed viable.

The financial criteria were intended to identify companies that not only were considered outstanding by industry leaders but also were financially strong. Consequently, we adopted as criteria for selection four measures of viability identified by the *1983 Investor's Guide To Health Maintenance Organizations*. We also used the data base from that study, which includes four years of statistics on the nation's 60 largest HMOs. The criteria for selection were:

— Average annual enrollment growth rate

— Return on sales (after-tax net income divided by premium revenue)

— Operating margin (premium revenue minus benefit expenditures, divided by premium revenue)

— The ratio of general and administrative expenses to total expenses

To be included in our study, an HMO must have ranked above the average for at least three of the four years and showed a trend of improving results. Thus, it must have demonstrated enrollment growth and good financial performance.

The final step was to select from the group above HMOs representing a mix of different service delivery models and organizational types. We also had to accept the reality that participation was voluntary on the part of the HMOs and that, given the considerable demands of hosting a site visit team, some would just be too busy being successful to spare the time to be studied.

Definition of Terms*

HMOs are generally classified into one of four types, the distinguishing features of which relate to how participating physicians are organized and paid. The four types are as follows:

— *Staff.* Participating physicians are salaried employees of the HMO who provide most outpatient services at the plan's multispecialty ambulatory care center or centers. Only rarely do these physicians provide a significant volume of fee-for-service care, and any resulting income accrues to the HMO rather than to individual physicians.

---

* Readers familiar with HMO terminology may wish to skip this section.

— *Group.* Physician services are arranged for by contracting with an independent multispecialty group practice, whose members then become the plan's participating doctors. In some situations, the group practice predated the HMO and served only fee-for-service patients. The HMO pays the group a negotiated capitation, that is, a fixed sum per enrollee per month. Referrals to nonparticipating doctors are usually paid out of the capitation also. In addition, there may be a bonus plan to create an incentive for doctors to control hospital costs.

— *Independent Practice Association (IPA).* Rather than relying upon centralized group practices, the HMO, either directly or through a formally organized physician association, generally contracts with solo practitioners and small, typically single-specialty, groups. These HMOs commonly have large panels of participating physicians whose practice is mostly fee-for-service. Consumers are often attracted by easier access to primary care sites and the wider choice of physicians, which may include their present doctors.

— *Network.* Network models closely resemble group-model HMOs, except that the HMO contracts with two or more independent group practices. Each group receives capitation payments from the HMO for enrollees who designate that medical group. Most groups that are part of a network continue to serve fee-for-service patients. Increasingly, the groups in the network are either capitated for hospital as well as physician services or share heavily in the risk, subject to a stop-loss, or maximum liability (for example, $15,000 per patient), beyond which the HMO bears full responsibility.

Staff and group models are often referred to as *closed panel* because their physicians typically see only HMO patients. In contrast, IPA and network plans are *open panel,* because participating physicians have both HMO and fee-for-service patients. These distinctions are becoming blurred, however, as the health plans adapt to increasing competition by developing multiple products to offer consumers.

Any HMO may seek to become *federally qualified* under Title XIII of the Public Health Service Act by applying to the Office of Prepaid Health Care in the Health Care Financing Administration (previously the Office of HMOs in the Public Health Service). Federal qualification has both advantages and disadvantages. On the positive side, it is viewed as a seal of approval by some employers. Perhaps more important, only federally qualified HMOs can take advantage of the right to *mandate* employers under what is known as the dual-choice provision of the act. The law says that an employer with more than 25 employees must offer at least one closed-panel (staff or group) and one open-panel (IPA or network) HMO to employees if the HMOs are federally qualified, if they provide services in the appropriate geographic area, and if they request in writing to be offered. Some HMOs do not follow this process, in order to avoid antagonizing employers. Others decline to become federally qualified in order to retain greater flexibility, for example in their benefit package design and methods of setting rates.

Health maintenance organizations are paid by subscribers (or by employers on behalf of subscribers) on a prepaid, per capita basis. *Capitation* is a fixed payment per enrollee paid to the HMO, usually on a monthly basis. This method of payment puts the HMO *at risk* for the provision of health services covered in its contract with the payer. Many HMOs, in turn, pay some health care providers on a capitated basis. For example, it is common for network and group models to pay groups of physicians on a per capita basis, thus putting them at risk for physician services. Some IPAs pay individual physicians a per capita amount, and even hospitals are being capitated by some HMOs.

Overview of the HMOs Studied

The eight HMOs studied, all of which are federally qualified, include two networks, three IPAs, and three staff models. The plans are located in six different states (three of them in California). Three are part of multistate HMO firms. Three are for-profit, and five are nonprofit, although one nonprofit is operated by a for-profit management firm.

Bay Pacific Health Plan is a for-profit IPA-model HMO that served San Mateo, San Francisco, and Marin counties in California at the time of our site visit. The plan has since expanded into Contra Costa and Alameda counties, thus effectively blanketing the San Francisco Bay Area. It was originally nonprofit and was started in 1979 by about 200 physicians and four hospitals in San Mateo County to counter the loss of market share to Kaiser Health Plan. It subsequently formed separate IPAs in San Francisco and Marin counties. Membership has now reached 60,000, and the number of participating physicians (both primary care providers and specialists) has reached 1,800. Bay Pacific management formed a for-profit partnership in 1983 to create reserves and secure capital for expansion. In late 1984, Bay Pacific Health Corporation, a publicly held, for-profit corporation, was formed and immediately acquired the partnership and the health plan.

Capital Area Community Health Plan is a nonprofit HMO that serves about 83,000 members in the Albany region of New York, southwestern Vermont, and western Massachusetts. Founded in 1977 as a staff model in which all physicians were salaried employees, Capital Area has since entered into contracts with fee-for-service medical groups in some of the areas into which it has expanded. It also has established HMOs in three small communities in western Massachusetts as joint ventures with the community hospitals there. The plan was started in large part from a conviction that HMOs can function successfully in rural areas, and several of its delivery sites are clinics staffed by two to three primary care physicians in small communities in New York and Vermont. The medical staff consists of 70 full-time and 20 part-time physicians in New York and Vermont: the Massachusetts joint ventures involve 26 primary care physicians and 70 specialists affiliated with the participating hospitals.

Harvard Community Health Plan (HCHP) is a nonprofit staff-model HMO with over 200,000 members. The plan was initiated by Harvard Medical School in 1969 and operates as an independent corporation. It has eight health centers, with two more under development, and serves five counties in greater Boston. The plan employs nearly 300 salaried physicians and almost 200 midlevel providers. It uses its own hospital for some nontertiary services and contracts with 14 other hospitals. A large proportion of admissions is to hospitals that are affiliated with Harvard University.

HMO of Pennsylvania (HMO-PA) is a proprietary IPA-model plan that is owned and operated by U.S. Healthcare. Established as a holding company subsequent to the initial success of HMO-PA, U.S. Healthcare operates HMOs in five states. Founded in 1977, HMO-PA now has 340,000 enrollees and serves seven counties in the Philadelphia and Allentown areas. The plan was one of the first IPAs in the country to successfully capitate individual primary care physicians. It capitates 560 such physicians for most services. In addition, each primary care physician has targets for hospital and specialty care and faces strong financial incentives to be judicious in the use of referral and inpatient care. HMO-PA contracts with 3,800 specialists and 62 hospitals.

Lifeguard HMO is a nonprofit IPA with 80,000 members. It grew out of the Santa Clara County Foundation for Medical Care and became operational in 1979. With headquarters in the Silicon Valley, the area around San Jose, it contracts with about 2,000 physicians in all specialties in four counties south and east of San Francisco. Physicians are paid on a fee-for-service basis, with 15 percent withheld from the maximum amount allowed by the fee schedule to cover budget overruns. Any overruns are shared by participating physicians in proportion to their contribution to the withholding pool. Fourteen contracted hospitals are used for inpatient care. Excess utilization is addressed largely through effective prior authorization and concurrent review programs for inpatient care and a sophisticated ambulatory claims review system.

Maxicare California is the original plan of Maxicare Health Plans, Inc. It started as a nonprofit HMO in 1973 but changed to for-profit status in 1980. Maxicare California serves 245,000 members from seven counties in Southern California, from Santa Barbara to San Diego. A network model, the plan contracts with over 30 medical groups and more than 50 community hospitals. It also operates its own hospital. Groups, most of which are multispecialty, are capitated for physician services, including referral care. The plan is at risk for hospital services but shares any surplus fifty-fifty with the medical group that generated it. Maxicare also has a new arrangement with 15 high-cost hospitals: the hospitals and their medical staffs are capitated for almost all services, but Maxicare provides administrative, marketing, and out-of-area services.

Rhode Island Group Health Association (RIGHA) is a nonprofit, staff-model plan that serves about 60,000 members in Rhode Island and southern Massachusetts. The plan was founded in 1971. Its labor origins created a strong community base, which the plan continues to cultivate. The plan employs over 60 salaried primary care physicians and specialists and also contracts with additional specialists. It has three health centers, and additional sites are being developed. About 75 percent of RIGHA's admissions are to hospitals affiliated with Brown University.

SHARE-Minnesota is a nonprofit, network-model HMO serving slightly more than 127,000 people in seven counties surrounding Minneapolis and St. Paul. It started as a staff model in 1974, and the medical group that comprised the original staff has 65 physicians at six locations. More recently, the HMO has entered into contracts with 25 group practices in areas not previously served; the 175 physicians in these groups now serve 55,000 of the members. The HMO also has contracts with 250 consulting specialists. In 1974 the senior management of SHARE-Minnesota formed SHARE Development Corporation, a for-profit entity that provides management services to SHARE-Minnesota under contract and has also established wholly owned, for-profit HMOs in several other states. In 1985 SHARE Development Company became part of United HealthCare Corporation, another large HMO firm, through an exchange of stock.

Site Visits

The field work for the project consisted of site visits to the eight HMOs between June 1984 and July 1985. Staff from Birch & Davis Associates, Inc. visited Bay Pacific, SHARE, and Capital Area, while staff from Lewin and Associates, Inc. visited HMO-PA, RIGHA, Lifeguard, and Maxicare. In a joint effort, one staff member from each firm visited HCHP.

Materials were collected from the HMOs beforehand. These were typically the annual report, resumes of top staff, marketing materials, a member handbook, the benefit package, provider contracts, and financial statements.

In most instances, a two-person team spent three days at each site. Interviews were set up by the HMO, using guidelines supplied by the team. The goal was to interview as many top managers as possible, including one or more board members, and to meet with operational staff in various functional areas (marketing, finance, provider relations, member services, and so on).

An interview guide helped structure the discussions, but it was not followed rigidly. The intent of the visits was to understand success through plan managers' eyes and to observe management style and corporate culture as well as actual practices and innovations. Seeing the marketing presentation to an employer or a group of Medicare beneficiaries, visiting HMO health centers and hospitals, and observing how the various functions related to one another were especially valuable.

The products of the site visits are case studies of each plan, four of which are included in this book. The case studies were reviewed by the HMOs in draft form to ensure accuracy and prevent the release of confidential information.

3

External Success Factors

Our major focus is on the internal operations of the HMOs studied. Nonetheless, various factors in the external environment are generally viewed as facilitating success. In this chapter we discuss how some of the HMOs appear to have been influenced by selected factors, including early entry into the market, the demographics of the community, the structure of the local insurance industry, and provider supply characteristics. (For a review of literature related to internal and external factors of success in HMOs, see the appendix.)

In most of the HMOs we studied, early entry into the market contributed to growth and protected market share. Lifeguard, for example, was the first IPA with a broad physician base in Santa Clara County, as was Bay Pacific in San Mateo County immediately to the north, although Kaiser, a group-model HMO, has been in the market for a number of years. Many observers believe that Kaiser stimulates IPA development as a competitive response on the part of fee-for-service physicians and that it educates the communities it serves about prepayment. Although concerned about new and potentially formidable competitors, Dorothy Emerson, executive vice president of Lifeguard, commented, "We have the product [that is, the broad physician network] and they don't."

Similarly, RIGHA and HCHP were the first in their respective communities and were able to establish themselves before facing tough competition. As the initial entrants, they could make some mistakes along the way in a more forgiving milieu than today's. However, HCHP had difficulty penetrating the suburbs because of its reliance on expensive teaching hospitals; it now relies more heavily on community hospitals, allowing it to reduce premiums for suburban residents. Capital Area remains the only HMO in Albany and the rural counties that surround it.

Several plans in Los Angeles predated Maxicare, but Maxicare was the first to be federally qualified, and it moved aggressively to create a broad provider network and to mandate employers under Title XIII. Similarly, HMO-PA, now the largest IPA in the nation, was not the first in the Philadelphia area, which the prevailing wisdom held was inhospitable to HMO growth. However, HMO-PA president Leonard Abramson described that perspective as "the prevailing excuse," and the plan became the first to establish a broad provider network and to market aggressively. Thus, neither Maxicare nor HMO-PA was the first in its community. Their success resulted from a willingness to capitalize on opportunities in the face of what must have appeared to be long odds. The theme of focusing on opportunity is developed further in chapter 6; the major point here is that success resulted from a combination of the presence of opportunities and the ability to capitalize upon them.

During its rapid growth phase in the late 1970s, SHARE faced considerable competition from larger, well-established plans. It was the first in its area to be federally qualified, however, and it made extensive use of the federal mandate in marketing to employers.

Early market entry was facilitated in some cases by the availability of federal funding under Title XIII. Between 1975 and 1980, all eight plans received either grants or loans from the Office of HMOs or its predecessor agency, both in the U.S. Department of Health and Human Services. Six plans (all but Bay Pacific and Lifeguard) were grant recipients. Capital Area and HCHP received grant funding in excess of $2 million each, while the other four received between $312,000 and $1.6 million. In addition, six plans (all but HCHP and Maxicare) obtained loans. These ranged from $747,000 in the case of Lifeguard to $2.5 million for HMO-PA.

Demographic and socioeconomic factors did little to explain the success of the HMOs studied. Even where these variables were statistically significant, the relationships were typically weak. There are numerous reasons for this lack of explanatory power. First, each of the HMOs encompasses a broad geographic area that includes populations with different levels of income and education. Other factors that are thought to affect HMO growth, such as unemployment, can change over time. (For example, both the Boston and the Los Angeles areas have been through cycles of unemployment over the last decade, although they are now doing well because of their high technology and defense industry base.) Population growth and the presence of multispecialty group practices have also been viewed as conducive to HMO growth, yet both HMO-PA and Capital Area have thrived in communities that lack these characteristics.

The structure of indemnity insurance exerted an influence on growth, but not a dominant one. Lifeguard executives feel that the prevalence of self-insurance in their area hurts them, both because the HMO in effect competes with the employer and because self-insured employers often have limited benefits, resulting in large premium contributions for employees who elect the HMO.

The presence of a Blue Cross plan that pays hospitals considerably below full charges (often by 20 percent or more) can be a more formidable threat. RIGHA has handled the problem by contracting with the Rhode Island Blue Cross Plan for claims processing, which enables RIGHA to pay hospitals at the lower rates. Now that RIGHA is larger, it is reassessing this arrangement. At first, HMO-PA overcame the price disadvantage by introducing physician reimbursement incentives and instituting tight controls on inpatient care in a community with high utilization. As it grew, its purchasing power increased, and it is now able to negotiate reimbursement levels that approximate those paid by the local Blue Cross plan. On the other hand, because most Blue Cross plans cover many services in full, that is, without patient cost sharing, they tend to charge high premiums. This creates a price umbrella for the HMO, an umbrella that is beginning to offer less protection now that there are more HMOs and other alternative delivery systems competing against one another.

The provider structure in the service areas of the HMOs has facilitated growth. All but one of the plans are in communities with an ample supply of physicians. (The exception is Capital Area, one of whose missions is to serve rural areas.) Certainly for the physicians associated with the five IPA or network models studied, the desire to protect patient volume stimulated participation in the plan and generated a willingness to accept its philosophy and operating procedures. Hospital utilization is high in all the service areas of the plans except California, where lower-than-average utilization may reflect the long-standing presence of Kaiser and Ross-Loos (now part of CIGNA).

Clearly, the national trend toward adoption of cost management measures, combined with the support of government, has created fertile soil for HMO growth. What emerges on balance, however, is that external factors do little to explain why the HMOs studied have been so successful. Thus fertile soil alone is not the cause of success—it is the way in which these plans have cultivated the soil, the subject of the next three chapters, that has made the difference.

4

Marketing and Consumer Relations

Health care is a service industry, and all of the HMOs studied exhibited strong and explicit service-oriented values. These values assume increasing importance as competition intensifies.

Service begins with the initial approach to employers. Federally qualified HMOs have an advantage enjoyed by few other services or products—namely, the mandate in Title XIII of the Public Health Service Act that employers offer HMOs (under defined circumstances) to employees. Several of the HMOs studied (for example, Maxicare, SHARE, HMO-PA) have aggressively used that federal mandate. However, Title XIII is intended only to foster fair marketplace competition; it does not require that anyone enroll or, once enrolled, remain with a plan.

As a result, the HMO needs to be responsive to the marketplace in at least three ways. First, it must persuade the employer that the firm and the employees will benefit, since employer attitudes, including the willingness to allow the HMO's marketing staff access to employees, have a strong bearing on ultimate enrollment. Second, it must persuade employees to enroll. Third, it must keep its customers satisfied after the sale. As a representative of HMO-PA said to us, word of mouth is the most important form of advertising. The HMOs studied make a point of serving employers after the sale and make it easy for members to use the system, have questions answered, and bring problems to the plan's attention. Efforts to maintain good relations with employers and members not only solve individual problems but also constitute sources of feedback on both the performance of individual providers and the acceptability of plan practices.

In this chapter we first discuss marketing, then consumer relations.

Marketing

The marketing of any product requires that attention be paid to product design, promotion, pricing, and selling or distribution. In this regard, HMOs are no different from any other enterprise; it is how they conduct these functions that is of interest.

In Touch with the Marketplace

All of the HMOs we studied exhibit *a commitment to being accepted in the marketplace.* This entails a continuous process of obtaining information on customer preferences and adapting the product to meet new challenges and opportunities.

All of the HMOs make conscious efforts to disperse delivery sites throughout their service areas in order to be geographically convenient to potential enrollees. For Bay Pacific and Lifeguard, reliance on fee-for-service physicians in the community ensured broad and geographically dispersed physician participation from the start. Others have had to make more conscious efforts. For example, RIGHA, a staff model that until recently delivered ambulatory services at a single location, is opening up roughly two sites a year to ring the city of Providence. In addition to the eight health centers it currently has, HCHP is committed to two more and is planning for an additional five. To avoid gaps in its delivery network, HMO-PA actively recruits primary care physicians in targeted locations around Philadelphia. One function of the marketing staff at SHARE is to identify areas where medical groups should be recruited.

Maxicare solicited the participation of group practices in the Palmdale and Lancaster areas in the desert, remote from their Los Angeles base, principally to serve employees of Rockwell International. Capital Area in Albany has expanded to 16 centers in upstate New York, Vermont, and western Massachusetts. Bay Pacific expanded from its original service area of San Mateo County to San Francisco and Marin counties by establishing new IPAs and is now expanding throughout Northern California. These expansions reflect more than simply seeking to attract new employer groups, they also represent an effort to match the residential and commuting patterns of existing groups.

Achieving this dispersion of sites often involves adopting new modes of delivery, in some cases modifying longstanding traditions, particularly in the case of staff models. Capital Area, a staff model, developed a series of small satellites with as few as three primary care doctors in rural areas of upstate New York. It then affiliated with multispecialty group practices under risk contracts and created joint ventures with small community hospitals. HCHP performs careful site selection studies and also contracts with some community physicians on a capitated basis to provide specialty services in its health centers. Maxicare, traditionally a network model that contracts with multispecialty groups, has started to capitate hospitals and their medical staffs in order to attract additional enrollees in parts of Los Angeles. Under this program, each hospital and medical staff receives a predetermined percentage of the premium for each enrollee and is responsible for providing or paying for essentially all medical care. This program, as well as a similar but more limited program at HMO-PA, was designed to protect the HMO financially by shifting virtually all of the financial risk to providers. Doing so makes it feasible to contract with prestigious but expensive hospitals.

There are many other examples of how HMOs respond to consumers. The physical appearance of the office is important, and many of the plans pay attention to office decor and patient flow. Maxicare and HMO-PA both assess the attractiveness of the medical offices of physicians before contracting with them.

RIGHA asks that enrollees sign up with a primary care physician, who serves as case manager, but it does not rigidly enforce this practice; indeed, it has provisions for walk-in services. Managing the costs of referral care was a consideration in instituting this policy, but another objective was to dispel the clinic image by emphasizing that each enrollee has a personal physician.

Some employers have complained about inflexibility, or lack of choice, in HMO benefit packages. Maxicare has made an effort to enhance employer choice by creating a variety of options for services covered and levels of copayment.

Several of the HMOs (for example, Maxicare, Capital Area, and HMO-PA) emphasize wellness programs as a marketing tool, and Maxicare offers free classes—for example, smoking cessation, weight reduction, and stress management—to all employees of some of its employer groups, not just to those employees who enroll in the plan. This differentiates them from the competition, emphasizes their commitment to wellness, and makes enrollment attractive to employees who are not members.

Finally, several of the HMOs we visited are developing related products, such as preferred provider organizations (PPOs) or utilization review services, that draw on the plans' provider networks and cost management skills. SHARE is developing a PPO, and Bay Pacific, through its new PPO subsidiary, intends to market an array of products in response to changing demands of group purchasers. These products would allow patients to use nonparticipating providers if they wanted to, but those who did would face higher cost sharing in the form of deductibles and coinsurance. Maxicare has created a subsidiary, HealthCare Alternatives, to perform utilization review for large employers, although it has only a limited number of contracts. Maxicare also recently purchased an insurance company. The parent company of HMO-PA, U.S. Healthcare, had announced plans to undertake a series of joint ventures, including HMO and PPO development, with Lincoln National Insurance Company. However, the relationship was subsequently terminated. Both RIGHA and Lifeguard are considering whether to market commercially their utilization review and HMO management computer software packages. A staff model, HCHP, is learning about IPA management through Managed Care, a for-profit firm that was started by HCHP and involved the movement of four senior staff to the new firm. Lifeguard has also formed an IPA management firm, IPA-USA.

The next few years are likely to witness more aggressive moves into new product lines. Meanwhile, in the current environment of rapid growth, the plans are by and large concentrating their energies on increasing their enrollment. Many of them are expanding into other states rather than diluting management talent by developing new, albeit closely related, product lines, although there are some indications that this trend may be changing.

The HMOs studied know their marketplace, have made conscious decisions regarding the populations they wish to attract, and have aggressive strategies for growth. All of the HMOs target large employers, both public and private. Lifeguard focuses only on firms with more than 100 employees and will generally not accept firms with fewer than 50. All of the plans market to Taft-Hartley trust funds,[1] although Lifeguard and Maxicare have not made them a high priority. In contrast, RIGHA, reflecting in part the strong role that labor leaders have played as founders and board members, has a specialist whose major function is to market to unions.

Not all of the HMOs accept employers with fewer than 25 employees or market to individual enrollees other than those covered by Medicare. However, HCHP now targets these small groups, and SHARE has actively marketed to nongroup enrollees. RIGHA accepts individual enrollees (subject to a medical screen) and finds this group to be financially profitable. Capital Area has from its inception enrolled groups with as few as four employees; in rural areas, it accepts individual enrollees.

All of the plans were at the very least seriously considering entering into a Medicare risk contract. The most aggressive has been SHARE, which has one of the highest Medicare enrollments (35,000) of any HMO in the country. Most of these persons enrolled under the demonstration contract that preceded the 1982 Medicare amendments. Maxicare signed a risk contract in California after a successful experience in Illinois, though it is increasingly questioning its Medicare relationship. Although some plans have hesitated to enter the Medicare market, the desire to grow in order to meet heightened competition makes it inevitable that most will do so. Similarly, small group and nongroup enrollment is likely to become more attractive as the larger groups become saturated.

All of the plans have underwriting standards similar to those that indemnity carriers apply before covering small employers. These standards determine the groups that the HMO will not actively market to because the financial risks are viewed as excessive, for example industries that have histories of heavy use of health services. Some HMOs also avoid firms whose employer contribution to premiums is so low that employees face a high differential if they join the HMO, potentially leading to adverse selection.

Finally, *some of the plans, recognizing that HMO enrollment is not for everyone, express the desire not to oversell, in order to avoid generating unrealistic expectations among enrollees.* This creates a problem in rewarding the sales force. Maxicare and HMO-PA discourage overpromising by tightly structuring the sales presentations of their marketing representatives. Other

HMOs pay their marketing representatives a straight salary and avoid commissions (or keep them low), consciously accepting the reduced motivation to increase enrollment. There is also concern that high bonuses can result in sales representatives' withholding information needed by the underwriting department to identify high-risk groups that should be denied coverage. (HMO-PA and Bay Pacific seek to avoid this problem by keeping the underwriting and sales functions separate.)

Lifeguard avoids sales commissions and reports that it does not want the sales force to come across as "too salesy." RIGHA introduced bonuses recently, but they are low. HCHP introduced a group bonus for the entire marketing staff if membership growth targets are met, reasoning that individual bonuses generate excessively strong incentives. In contrast, HMO-PA, Bay Pacific, and SHARE establish quotas and compensate their sales force primarily through commissions.

A Carefully Structured Approach to Employers and Employees

Most of the HMOs have a highly organized, well-managed approach to selling that leaves little to chance. Marketing representatives are assigned geographic territories. HMO-PA uses a separate staff to identify sales prospects, thus allowing marketing representatives to sell rather than conduct research on whom to approach. Employer contracts are synchronized with the organization's open enrollment or contract renewal periods, and followup protocols after both the initial contact and the sale are well developed. Some of the plans, such as HMO-PA and Maxicare, rely on computers to manage and track the marketing process, starting with the development of a list of initial prospects and running through to the point of sale.

Many of the plans (for example, Maxicare and HMO-PA) have a standard sales pitch, emphasizing the uniqueness of the product, to assure that a consistent message is delivered. Lifeguard, although less rigid in its approach, establishes themes that the marketing representatives rehearse while in training. Several plans (for example, HCHP, RIGHA, Maxicare) emphasize quality of care, in part to differentiate themselves from the competition. Other messages delivered by the plans stress wellness, having one's own physician, comprehensiveness of coverage, low and predictable out-of-pocket expenses, the lack of claims forms, and (particularly in the case of IPAs such as Lifeguard and Bay Pacific) access to a broad provider network.

Several plans alter their approaches when selling to non-group enrollees. SHARE has a large, highly successful telephone marketing program to attract individual and Medicare enrollees, and HCHP has done the same for its Medicare program. To generate Medicare enrollment, Maxicare and Bay Pacific sponsor community meetings at hospitals, senior citizen centers, and other places.

The professionalism of the sales force was notable in all of the plans. Maxicare hires only college graduates and describes their typical representative as "enthusiastic, smart, and career-oriented." All of the plans have training programs. Some of them are mostly on-the-job, whereas others are highly formalized, with lengthy sales manuals, role playing by trainees, and regular quizzes. The training programs address both how the plan functions and how to approach employers and employees. Some of the plans send marketing representatives to sales technique classes conducted by the Group Health Association of America. (These classes are modeled after the highly successful courses first developed by the Xerox Corporation.)

Advertising campaigns, principally on television and radio and in newspapers, have become critical in gaining popular recognition. Several of the HMOs (Maxicare, HMO-PA, SHARE) have been the first to advertise heavily in their respective markets. *The plans carefully select their advertising messages and symbols.* As with the marketing representatives' sales presentations, the advertising messages emphasize comprehensiveness of coverage, lack of claims forms, convenience of access to services, personal physicians, superior quality of care, and commitment to wellness and disease prevention. Maxicare intentionally does not mention the term "HMO" in its advertising; instead, given the limited information that can be conveyed, it stresses what the plan does for its enrollees.

Use is also made of slogans and symbols which emphasize that the plans care about the health of their members. The heart is the symbol of Lifeguard, and its slogan is "Lifeguard keeps you well." Bay Pacific's is "Your Partner in Good Health." HMO-PA uses a red apple on all of its advertising and brochures. Its sales representatives wear bright red blazers, as do actors in the television commercials, thereby achieving a consistent image in all communications. HMO-PA representatives also distribute apples at their initial presentations to employees. SHARE features the slogan, "There's so much more to SHARE."

All the plans recognize the importance of good service to employers after the sale. In some plans, such as Maxicare and HMO-PA, the marketing representatives provide the service. Maxicare also has a minimum number of callbacks, which varies by group size, that should be made to each employer. Staying in touch regularly is designed to spot problems before they become severe and to give employers the sense that they have someone to call upon. Other plans—such as SHARE, RIGHA, HCHP, Capital Area, and Bay Pacific—have separate staffs for providing service to employers, although in some cases they are located within the marketing department. These plans reason that service after the sale requires different skills than marketing, and they want to ensure that the employers receive adequate attention.

The sales force may also be a source of information for product improvements. For example, a benefits manager at Hughes Helicopter told a Maxicare marketing representative of his discontent with the plan's alcohol and drug abuse services, and the plan took measures to correct the situation.

Pricing Strategies

The HMOs differ in their pricing policies. Several, including Maxicare, Bay Pacific, RIGHA, Lifeguard, and HCHP, set premiums above those of their HMO competitors and emphasize in their marketing quality of care, access to care, or both. Others seek to have the lowest prices in the community, or nearly so. All the plans know what it costs per member to provide services, and they make sure that premiums are sufficient. Should their premiums exceed what the marketplace permits, they will reexamine their costs in order to bring revenues and expenses into line. This might entail assessing areas where utilization can be further reduced or negotiating better reimbursement arrangements with providers.

Almost all of the plans are feeling more intense price competition and have reacted by keeping premium increases below past levels. This reflects both competition from other HMOs and cost management initiatives among indemnity plans. In its budgeting process for the current year, HCHP has made restraining costs a major priority. The plan is trying to control hospital costs by directing volume to providers with whom favorable terms have been negotiated. A new IPA competitor with low premiums and broad benefits forced RIGHA to reduce its annual rate of premium increase to 3 percent in 1985, compared to 14 percent in 1981 and 1982 and 9 percent in 1983.[2] At the same time, RIGHA has sought to improve its utilization data in order to identify opportunities for reducing hospital use. In addition to restraining premium increases, Bay Pacific is introducing multiple benefit programs that allow the employer to elect higher cost sharing in return for lower premiums.

Another tactic for keeping prices competitive is to vary premiums by geographic areas. For example, HCHP introduced a separate, lower premium structure in the suburbs of Boston because a premium structure reflecting the use of expensive downtown teaching hospitals placed it at a competitive disadvantage in those communities.

Interestingly, none of the HMOs we visited has availed itself of the full flexibility in premium setting—known as community rating by class—that federal law permits. Community rating by class entails varying the rates charged each group to reflect such objective factors as enrollee age and type of industry. Some argue that this flexibility allows HMOs to approximate the experience rating practices of indemnity insurers. Instead, the plans use community rating, with only minor variations. One plan president said, tongue in cheek, that HMOs are not sophisticated enough to do anything more complex. More to the point, strict community rating has the advantage of simplicity in an era of rapid expansion. Pricing is facilitated, and the large actuarial and underwriting staffs that characterize the typical insurance company can be avoided. Also, complex rating structures can make plans more vulnerable to having to negotiate premiums with employers. Several HMOs said that they are reassessing their premium-setting practices in the face of increasing competition and pressures from employers, which may force them to adopt more refined pricing mechanisms.

Consumer Relations

Health care is a product steeped in emotion. Although quality of care is difficult for consumers to assess, the way they are treated by an organization is not. The member services or consumer relations department is an important link between the HMO and its ultimate customer. *It is a vehicle for answering consumer ques-*

tions and a vital source of feedback to plan management on providers' performance. Some plans use the department to track problems, to find aspects of the health plan that are problematic or confusing to members, or both. By using consumer relations in this way, the plan is often able to turn a complaint into a positive interaction, that is, into an opportunity to serve an individual member or to improve the plan. Word of mouth is a powerful marketing tool, hence satisfied customers are a valuable asset, particularly in an era of increased competition.

Investment of Resources in People and Systems

One characteristic of many plans is that they have not stinted on resources: instead, *they have hired sufficient staff and have developed training programs, job requirements, and performance standards to ensure a high level of customer service.*

Maxicare, for example, hires only college graduates as consumer affairs representatives, and all of them participate in a formal, three-week training program. The plan has one representative per approximately 8,000 members, which is a relatively high staffing ratio. HMO-PA trains specialized complaint researchers to work in areas where problems typically occur, such as enrollment and claims. The plan has also developed consistent answers to commonly asked questions: these answers are circulated in memos to all staff who encounter the public.

The telephone is a major tool of consumer relations, and many plans have been innovative in using it. While not part of consumer affairs, HMO-PA's telephone marketing staff perform a customer service by calling all new members to welcome them to the plan and answer any questions. HMO-PA has invested in computerized telephone systems, similar to those used by airlines, which automatically record caller-waiting times and divert calls to available representatives. Lifeguard is investigating the possibility of installing an automated response center that would allow members to call for taped answers to their questions at any time of the day or night.

As another example of the investment in consumer relations, Bay Pacific annually sends its entire enrollment a membership satisfaction survey. Results are reflected in changes in benefits or plan operations. Bay Pacific has also instituted a program of calling members in selected accounts 90 days before open enrollment to discuss satisfaction with the HMO.

Strong Service Orientation

The HMOs have devised creative ways of ensuring member access to physicians and nurses throughout the plan and of improving service. HMO-PA makes regular, unannounced checks on primary care physicians by calling their offices on weekends and in the evening. If the response time is over 30 minutes on two attempts, the physician is informed that he or she is in violation of plan standards and may ultimately be disciplined. The plan also requires that physicians have beeper systems that enable them to be contacted when they are away from the office. HCHP regularly conducts checks to see how quickly phones are answered at various locations throughout the plan. Lifeguard consumer representatives give their names and invite members to call back with any further problems they may encounter; in addition, calls are divided alphabetically to promote continuity.

Many plans actively encourage the airing of complaints because they want to know if members are unhappy. To facilitate this, both Maxicare and HMO-PA provide members with grievance forms. Maxicare and Capital Area have representatives at several employer locations to improve access for members, allow face-to-face contact, and defuse problems early. Maxicare consumer representatives can authorize payment of claims of up to $100 for walk-in or telephone problems; the plan believes this contributes to the morale of representatives as well as to member satisfaction.

Information from Consumer Relations as a
Source of Feedback

Consumer relations can be a significant source of feedback to management on plan performance. In addition to solving problems and answering questions as they arise, consumer relations staff serve as a source of information to the plan as a whole. *Many HMOs have formal or informal procedures to classify the nature of calls, report this information to other managers, and follow up with corrective strategies.*

RIGHA incorporates consumer complaints into its quality assurance process: for example, it has redesigned its telephone appointment system in response to complaints about access. Lifeguard uses member complaints as a source of information about possibly inappropriate care by physicians. The plan's consumer relations staff views itself as the hub of a wheel, performing an integrative function across all departments. HMO-PA uses consumer relations to determine where problems exist in the health service delivery system; it tracks all complaints by category, disseminates the results, and makes adjustments accordingly. For example, if new members are unhappy with the HMO's lock-in, under which services provided by non-HMO providers are not covered, the sales pitch of marketing representatives will be reexamined to be sure they are conveying the requirement that all care must be delivered by HMO-sanctioned providers. HMO-PA also surveys a sample of patients from each primary care physician's panel as part of its annual recertification process. HCHP surveys a sample of its members every two months, tabulates about 20 measures of member satisfaction separately for each health center, and watches trends closely. One change it made in response to member feedback was to increase monitoring of telephone calls in order to catch problems early and reduce waiting times. Member preference for small health centers has also been a factor in the plan's moving to smaller centers.

Attention from Top Management

As described above, many HMOs prepare summary reports for management describing the types of calls received from members. These reports often receive top-level attention. For example, RIGHA's medical director personally reviews most complaints, and the chief executive officer (CEO) of U. S. Healthcare (HMO-PA's parent company) frequently visits the HMO-PA member services department. The CEO of Bay Pacific receives a monthly summary of complaints, and the board receives a quarterly summary. Maxicare's president receives a monthly summary of all complaints, classified by type of problem, and the regional medical director sees all complaints related to medical care. This attention from senior management is another guarantee that the HMO will be both responsive to member needs and able to adjust to the market.

Notes

1. It is common in certain industries, such as construction, where employees change jobs frequently, for the employer to make payments to a trust fund that is jointly managed by union and management repre-

sentatives in lieu of offering benefits directly. The Taft-Hartley bill, enacted in 1947, regulates these funds.

2. Some of this reduction reflects lower rates of inflation in the economy as a whole, but not all of it by any means. RIGHA is assessing whether the marketplace will sustain even 3 percent increases.

5

Provider Relations

In addition to having effective cost management, successful HMOs must have accessible, high-quality physicians. Physicians are largely responsible for an HMO's reputation in the community, and how they are selected, organized, and paid helps define the HMO. All health plans need a strategy for bringing physicians close to the organization and for involving them in the business so that they internalize the competitive goals of the plan. A combination of "psychology and behavior modification," in the words of one executive, is the most effective method. Physician leaders and managers play a major role in implementing this strategy by brokering the relationship between physicians and the plan.

A natural tension arises from HMOs' dual role as providers of care and insurers who are financially at risk; yet the HMOs in our study display an ability to balance the requirements of service delivery and cost management. Utilization of services can be controlled in a number of ways. One strategy is to select physicians with efficient practice patterns; however, the plans report that their ability to do this is limited. Rather, they rely on a combination of the following:

— Financial incentives

— Administrative controls over utilization of services

— The fostering of behavioral change among physicians through education and the promotion of an organizational culture

Most plans pursue more than one of these strategies, although there are variations by model type. For example, IPAs, which involve loose associations of individual practitioners, will rarely be able to instill an organizational culture that is as strong as that of a closed-panel plan, in which physicians are in daily contact with one another. Similarly, the use of financial incentives may clash with the culture of staff models such as RIGHA and HCHP but be more acceptable in a proprietary network that contracts with independent physicians or medical groups.

A common feature of all the plans is the recognition of a need for communication and education. Of particular concern is physician understanding of utilization statistics. Physicians must be cognizant of the impact of high utilization—including excess referrals to specialists and use of laboratory and X-ray services—on cost. This holds true even in plans where the physicians are heavily at risk, such as HMO-PA and SHARE, because physicians who are losing money are not likely to stay with the plan or continue providing high-quality care. Communication must be two-way, however, and many of the plans rely on clinicians for information about what is happening in the delivery system or in the local environment.

In this chapter we discuss four aspects of HMO-provider relations:

— The role of physicians and hospitals, notably how they are selected and the nature of their relationship to the HMO
— Provider reimbursement, focusing on risk sharing and financial incentives
— Utilization control
— Quality assurance

Physicians and Hospitals

In all of the HMOs studied, relations with physicians are the starting point for the delivery system. In most of them, primary care physicians are especially critical. At HCHP and RIGHA, hospitals are also an integral part of the plan, whereas at HMO-PA they are viewed more as contractors. Other plans fall in between on this spectrum.

The way in which physicians are selected, the leadership
they exert, their involvement in plan management, and the nature of relations with hospitals are highlighted in this section.

Physician Selection

*The process of selecting physicians is important to most of the
plans we visited, although some have more structured approaches
than others.* The process is always somewhat subjective, and self-
selection by physicians occurs as well. Reflecting the increase in
supply of physicians in recent years, all of the HMOs face a buyer's market for physician services and can afford to be selective.
This was not always the case, however; both HMO-PA and Capital Area, for example, encountered recruiting difficulties in their
early years.

Those HMOs that do select physicians carefully look for different attributes and establish their recruitment criteria accordingly. Some look for knowledge and understanding of prepaid
group practice. For example, RIGHA requires physician candidates to be interviewed twice at the plan so that their knowledge
and attitudes about HMOs can be fully explored; it also checks
references carefully. HCHP pays particular attention to academic
background and ability to obtain privileges at prestigious teaching
hospitals. Others require board eligibility and review credentials
but are more concerned with the location, accessibility, and aes-
thetic appeal of the office. Maxicare recruits high-quality medical
groups with strong reputations in the community; lengthy applications are required, and every facility must pass a precontract
review that includes two site visits. Maxicare says it seriously reviews fewer than one in ten applications received.

HMO-PA believes that selecting physicians carefully in the
first place is easier than firing poor performers later. The plan
seeks to recruit primary care physicians with an active hospital
practice because it has found that such physicians are more confi-
dent of their medical skills and therefore make fewer referrals
than physicians without a significant hospital practice. HMO-PA
visits the office of each applicant to examine record keeping, appointment scheduling, and physical appearance; the plan will not,
for example, hire a physician who schedules more than five or six
intermediate visits per hour. In addition, one of the HMO's medical directors interviews each applicant. One purpose of the interview is to assess the applicant's attitude; for example, the plan

prefers to reject physicians who are angry about HMO development but feel they must join in order to protect their practice.
HMO-PA denies 20 to 40 percent of primary care physician applicants, and those accepted are on conditional status for the first
two years. Capital Area, SHARE, HCHP, and Bay Pacific also
place new physicians on probation.

Although some plans feel they cannot survive without carefully selecting their physicians, this is not universally true. As is
typical of provider-sponsored IPAs, Lifeguard and Bay Pacific will
accept any physician who is a member in good standing of the local medical society. Although membership is now closed, Lifeguard used to accept physicians on a first come, first served basis.
One of Bay Pacific's IPAs now charges a $3,000 participation fee
and has a waiting list.

The IPA-model HMO serves a marketing function for physicians and can become an ongoing source of revenue, a fact that
plans stress in recruiting. However, according to one plan executive, it takes two years before a physician fully embraces the
HMO, understands its operating principles, and realizes what it
can do for his or her practice.

Physicians in Leadership Roles

Typically, one or more physicians are key members of the management team. In addition, physicians who have been with the
plan a long time, sit on the board, or who are widely respected by
their peers are often solicited by management for advice and for
their ability to lead other physicians. Most of the plans believe
that a highly placed and visible physician, usually the medical director, is important so that rank-and-file physicians can interact
with one of their own.

Physicians are generally more integrated into all levels of
management in group- and staff-model HMOs. Many of the older
HMOs are group or staff models, and they have an ideological
commitment to the group practice of medicine, including an emphasis on peer review and collaboration as opposed to the independence of the individual practitioner. In physician- or hospital-
sponsored IPAs and networks, physicians often play a dominant
role in policymaking, although not necessarily in daily management activities. In entrepreneurial plans, which are financed
heavily by outside investors, there is a tendency for authority to
be vested in a management team that includes one or more physi-

cians but that has more nonphysician input. This may result when the HMO sees itself as a business enterprise that provides health services rather than as a community-based health care provider that must remain financially viable.

Some of the qualities sought in physician leaders include (1) a practicing primary care physician who commands the respect of his or her peers, (2) an understanding of the HMO business and the competitive environment, (3) a belief that some controls on medical practice make sense, and (4) a readiness to confront colleagues about their practice patterns. Some plans report difficulty in finding physicians who are willing to confront other physicians on utilization issues.

The plans all have physician leaders who serve as interpreters and educators of other physicians and management. The position is one of a broker to some extent, since the most effective physician leaders are those who can communicate physicians' ideas and concerns to management and business needs to physicians. Highlighting the importance of communication, several plans report that physicians and nurses are the source of most innovation, such as new ways of reducing utilization.

Physician managers must walk a fine line, and at SHARE and HCHP several reported that they are sometimes seen by fellow physicians as having been co-opted by management. *Maintaining credibility as a physician is one reason some plans strongly encourage managers and medical directors to continue their clinical practices.* At HCHP, it is unspoken policy that every physician with management responsibilities, including the medical director, sees patients. In most of the plans, physician leaders (and their strength as perceived by other plan physicians) are important in recruiting new medical staff as well as in negotiating payment issues and other policies. Such leaders also act as troubleshooters, initiating contact and discussion with physicians who become restless or disillusioned with the plan.

Clinicians may have different objectives from managers, further underscoring the need for physician leadership. In most cases, the rewards for physicians are different from those for managers. For example, physicians, generally do not relish growth. Yet from the viewpoint of most managers and investors, a growing organization is a healthy one. Growth in a staff model can mean more crowding for physicians, tighter scheduling, and slower service from ancillary providers. In an IPA, growth can have a positive effect if the result is greater patient volume, but it can also generate greater competition among IPA physicians if more physicians are recruited. Similar disparities can arise on other issues, ranging from benefit package design (patient need as perceived by physicians versus market demand as perceived by managers) to hospital selection (convenience to physicians versus cost to plan). A successful physician leader accepts the need to mediate and communicate among the various parties.

The plans understand that physicians are trained to be highly individualistic and self-reliant and that they are not easily herded. In addition, the expectations most physicians acquired during the course of their training, in terms of both income and practice style, are often at variance with the reality of medical practice today. As a result, plans need a strategy for bringing physicians close to the organization so that they can accept and internalize its goals. The strategies employed by the plans are diverse. For example, HMO-PA uses psychology and behavior modification. It communicates constantly with its primary care physicians, educates them about cost-effective care, and assists them in organizing their practice, hiring new associates, and tracking performance. Subtle behavior modification occurs as physicians benefit financially from practicing efficiently.

At HCHP, in contrast, physicians are given full responsibility for managing health centers; thus their performance as managers becomes critical to the plan's viability. HCHP has strengthened its commitment to physician managers and invests heavily in training. Several physicians in high administrative positions have attended executive training programs at Harvard and Stanford business schools at the plan's expense. Besides a planwide medical director (one of two senior executives who share responsibility for overall plan management with the president), each of the eight health center directors is a physician who has line responsibility for all health care functions. This unusual practice is expensive and reflects HCHP's commitment to physician responsibility and accountability.

At both RIGHA and Capital Area, also staff models, the executive director and the medical director have a close working relationship and are often perceived as equals. In rural centers, Capital Area's medical directors fill the executive director role as well and have complete authority over operations. At RIGHA, each health center is run jointly by an associate medical director and an associate administrator.

At Lifeguard and Bay Pacific, both provider-based IPAs, physicians are heavily represented on the board; the president of Lifeguard is a physician. Day-to-day management is in the hands of nonphysicians, however. At both HMO-PA and Maxicare, one of the top decision makers is a physician, but the physician perspective tends not to dominate HMO policy.

Valued Physician Relationships

Regardless of the role that physicians play in decision making, the HMOs view a win-win relationship as critical. Several of the plans said that keeping physicians happy contributes to member satisfaction. The plans also recognize that physicians could leave and take patients with them. Therefore they have established processes for responding to physician needs and complaints that are analogous to the consumer relations function. The open-panel (network and IPA) plans tend to invest staff and resources in provider relations and to treat physicians as they would clients. In staff models, where most physicians are employees rather than contractors, physicians are treated more as colleagues than as clients. In these plans, responsiveness to physicians can be observed in the form of shared authority and physician involvement in decision making.

Some plans concern themselves mostly with primary care physicians, distinguishing between them and specialists. The most dramatic example in our study is HMO-PA, where primary care physicians are financially at risk and are responsible for coordinating all other medical services. These physicians receive a fixed monthly payment for the primary care of each enrollee in their panel and have strong financial incentives not to overuse specialist or hospital services. Because of the central role that these physicians play, the plan is both more careful in selecting them than they are in selecting specialists and more concerned that they be comfortable with the plan.

HMO-PA and Bay Pacific employ staff who train physicians' office employees to relate to the HMO. At HMO-PA, for example, physicians and their office managers are taught how to organize an HMO practice, including how to complete encounter forms (for recording patient visits) and how to interpret statistics showing how their utilization of services (for example, number of office visits, laboratory tests ordered, and hospitalization rates) compares with that of other physicians. HMO-PA also helps primary care physicians recruit new associates and improve their telephone systems. As another example, the medical groups with which Maxicare contracts are heavily at risk, but the plan offers assistance on such matters as how to compensate individual physicians within the group and how to conduct utilization review and quality assurance.

Compensation is an integral part of good relations with physicians. Under risk-sharing agreements, physicians are typically well compensated if the plan's financial objectives are met (HMO-PA, Maxicare, SHARE). Several plans stated that they try to ensure at least the equivalent of fee-for-service income for primary care physicians, even before any bonuses are paid. Similarly, Lifeguard's approach to maintaining good relations with physicians is to pay reasonable fees and to pay them promptly, usually within three to five days.

Relations with Hospitals

The HMOs we visited exhibited various attitudes toward their relations with hospitals, reflecting in part different perspectives on the importance of hospital affiliations in marketing and physician recruitment. HMO-PA believes that a hospital's location and willingness to negotiate on price are the most important criteria for affiliation: the company often identifies hospitals it wants to affiliate with and then accepts applications only from physicians who have privileges at those hospitals. Hospital relations as such, however, are not part of the plan's marketing strategy. Lifeguard views hospitals as secondary to physicians in terms of patient satisfaction. Neither plan markets its hospital affiliations or believes the use of teaching hospitals is important, except to recruit desirable physicians.

Hospitals are becoming more important players in some markets, especially when they assume financial risk. Maxicare is attempting to attract members who have not previously joined an HMO because of the limited physician and hospital choice. It recently began to capitate 15 prestigious hospitals in Southern California. These hospitals, along with their medical staffs, bear the risk for most aspects of patient care, in that each receives a fixed percentage of the premium for any member who elects to receive care from that hospital and medical staff. Since many of the hospitals are expensive, Maxicare can afford to contract with them only because they are willing to accept the financial risk. At the same time, the hospitals stand to gain if utilization is low.

Two of the staff-model plans in the study have used teaching hospitals extensively. RIGHA uses teaching hospitals affiliated with Brown University almost exclusively and views this relationship as important for marketing, consumer relations, and physician recruitment. The reliance of HCHP on university hospitals is a long-standing tradition and part of the plan's identity. The plan also has its own hospital and, concomitant with its expansion to the suburbs, has contracted with community hospitals near its suburban health centers. HCHP recently decided to solidify its relationship with one Harvard teaching hospital, Brigham and Women's Hospital. All HCHP physicians at health centers which use the Brigham will be given admitting privileges there, and deeply discounted rates have been negotiated for secondary care at the Brigham, rates that are roughly equal to costs in HCHP's own hospital.

Provider Reimbursement: Risk Sharing and Financial Incentives

HMOs have adopted a broad range of financial risk relationships with providers. These risk relationships have two principal dimensions. The first is the extent to which the HMO passes the risk along to providers, particularly to participating physicians. The second is the extent to which the incentives are collective or individualized; that is, whether large aggregations of providers gain or lose equally, based on their overall performance, or whether gain and loss are based on the performance of a single provider or small group of providers.

The HMOs in this study are able to operate successfully with different types of payment systems. Staff models such as RIGHA and HCHP tend to make less use of financial incentives than IPA and network plans. Provider-based IPAs such as Lifeguard are less inclined to institute risk sharing than entrepreneurial, investor-owned plans such as HMO-PA, SHARE, and Maxicare. *Most important, financial incentives and other methods of utilization control are designed jointly. What successful plans have in common is not a particular set of incentives, but a carefully constructed model that represents an appropriate mix of approaches to cost management.*

At first it might appear that capitating providers or otherwise requiring them to bear a high degree of risk would allow the

HMO to adopt a relaxed attitude toward utilization management. Such is not the case, for two reasons. First, if the providers fare poorly, they are prone to have negative attitudes toward HMO patients (thereby damaging member relations) and may ultimately cease to participate. Second, they are likely to pressure the plan to increase payment levels. This is particularly a problem when individual services, such as pharmacy and radiology, are capitated and then regarded almost as free by referring physicians. The HMOs in our study that have placed providers at risk have a tangible win-win philosophy under which they retain responsibility for the success of participating providers.

In our sample of HMOs, the financial incentives faced by physicians can be categorized as

— Fee-for-service
— Neutral (lack of incentives)
— Medical group at risk
— Individual physician at risk

Hospitals are typically not at risk, although competitive pressures are making them more interested in contracting with HMOs, including more interested in accepting risk. In some plans we studied, individual hospitals are partially at risk (such as through a withhold from fees), at risk for certain diagnoses (payment per case), or fully at risk (capitated).

Fee-for-Service Incentives

Many IPAs pay physicians fees for each item of service rendered. Typically, a percentage of the fee is withheld. This is not in itself a powerful incentive for controlling utilization, because the ultimate payment of the amount withheld is based on the performance of the plan as a whole and not on that of any one doctor. Consequently, other means of tracking and controlling utilization are necessary.

Lifeguard is a plan that pays on a fee-for-service basis. Fifteen percent of allowable fees is withheld to cover potential HMO budget overruns and is usually returned to physicians at six-month intervals. Some hospitals with which Lifeguard contracts are also subject to a risk withhold; these funds become part of the same pool as the physician withholds and are later returned if overall financial performance permits. No bonuses above 100 percent of allowable charges are generated.

Although Bay Pacific capitates its IPAs for physician services, individual physicians are paid negotiated fees, subject to a risk withhold of 20 percent for services provided in a hospital and 10 percent for those provided in a physician's office. Anything above the projected budget for out-of-plan referrals, ancillary services, and a portion of hospital care is charged against this risk pool. At the end of the year, the remainder is distributed to IPA-member physicians. Under the plan's Medicare risk contract, individual hospitals and their medical staffs receive a single capitation payment.

This method of payment adopted by Lifeguard and Bay Pacific serves to remind providers that they are not assured of full compensation if overall health services costs are excessive. The collective incentive to conserve, however, is more than offset by the individual incentive to provide services and be reimbursed on a fee-for-service basis. To counter this, Lifeguard and Bay Pacific have instituted tight utilization control mechanisms. The primary care physician serves as case manager and must authorize all referrals. The plans also require prior authorization for inpatient admissions and for many other procedures and services, have strong concurrent review, and have a sophisticated, computerized claims review system that results in regular scrutiny of physician practice profiles.

Neutral Incentives

Most staff model plans pay physicians a straight salary, which removes any fee-for-service incentive. Some plans also award bonuses based on planwide or health center performance.

At RIGHA, HCHP, and Capital Area, all staff models, most physicians are salaried and thus do not have direct financial incentives for altering their patterns of care. There are other motivations for controlling utilization, however. Budgets are carefully monitored at the department level, and managers disseminate utilization statistics. Indirect incentives exist, since funds for salary increases and bonuses depend on profitability. Careful selection of physicians and physician loyalty to the plan are clearly more important than these incentives. Further, staff-model plans create an environment in which interaction with peers and on-site specialists allows for more informal discussion of cases and, perhaps, fewer referrals.

A neutral incentive system does not encourage greater productivity, since compensation is not directly affected by volume of services provided. As a result, HCHP is experimenting with a new payment mechanism that provides incentives to improve productivity. Primary care physicians will be paid 85 percent of the normal salary for their specialty and seniority, with additional compensation accruing as a function of the number of members for whom they are responsible.

Medical Group Incentives

Providing incentives for medical groups involves placing the groups at risk to some degree. The physicians must then develop a strategy for payment and utilization control. For example, SHARE places physician group practices at risk for both physician and inpatient services. In the first three years of a group's contract, it shares surpluses equally with the plan; after that, 100 percent of the hospital budget surplus is returned to the group. Maxicare capitates its groups for physician services. For hospital services, it establishes expenditure targets for each group; Maxicare shares any surplus fifty-fifty but absorbs all losses. All of these arrangements include stop-loss provisions, which limit the financial risk associated with any individual patient.

Individualized Incentives

Perhaps the most powerful combination of incentives for individual physicians is capitation of primary care physicians combined with incentives to minimize use of specialists and inpatient care. Specialists, either individually or in small groups, are also capitated by some plans.

HMO-PA offers good examples of both. It capitates small primary care offices (usually one to five physicians) for primary care services and places them at risk for most of the cost of referrals to specialists. Targets are set for specialty services, and any surplus is paid in full to the primary care physician. Should the primary care physician face a loss, it is shared among all participating physicians. Primary care physicians are not at risk for radiology (other than simple X rays), laboratory, and mental health services, which the HMO capitates separately. Individual primary care physicians share hospital surpluses (relative to a target amount) equally with the HMO, while the HMO is at risk for hospital deficits.

To create countervailing pressures to assure that enrollees receive appropriate services, HMO-PA audits primary care physician practices and solicits consumer feedback. The plan audits every doctor's office annually, including examination of utilization statistics for evidence of underutilization and review of any complaints filed against the office. Underutilization is detected principally through an analysis of the encounter forms that physicians are required to complete for each patient visit. Finally, the plan makes patients and physicians aware that patients can switch physicians if they are dissatisfied.

Hospitals and Other Providers at Risk

Usually HMOs reimburse hospitals on either a negotiated per diem or a discounted charge basis. Both Maxicare and HCHP own a small hospital that they use for some secondary services and, in the case of HCHP, urgent and after-hours care. Nonetheless, the majority of hospital services is provided by community hospitals under contract.

Increasingly, HMOs are seeking to put hospitals at risk for all or some part of their services. Four of the plans have arrangements with selected hospitals to transfer financial risk. In some cases, the plans would not have used high-cost hospitals if capitation were not the mode of payment. The fact that so many well-regarded but expensive community and teaching hospitals are willing to accept risk also reflects heightened marketplace pressures.

Maxicare's Project Window in Southern California is the most ambitious attempt at hospital capitation. Fifteen prestigious teaching hospitals and their medical staffs (not known for conservative utilization patterns) are fully capitated for all physician and hospital services, excluding out-of-area coverage and a few other items. HMO-PA has also capitated two Philadelphia teaching institutions, a move initially prompted by the high utilization patterns of the associated medical faculty. Further, HMO-PA pays some hospitals on a per case basis: for 11 procedures that account for between 40 and 50 percent of admissions, the HMO has developed its own prospective payment system. The plan has, for example, achieved significant savings on admissions for normal delivery and open-heart surgery. Capital Area has entered into joint ventures with three small community hospitals in which the hospitals are at risk for inpatient costs. Bay Pacific has risk contracts with all the hospitals it uses in San Francisco and San Mateo.

Maxicare and HMO-PA also capitate community pharmacies, paying them a fixed amount per member per month to cover all prescription drugs used by HMO members. HMO-PA limits the pharmacy's risk by guaranteeing the costs of acquiring drugs should those costs exceed the agreed-upon capitation levels. At Maxicare, pharmacies are at full risk for prescriptions, but the plan provides them with considerable assistance to help them lower their costs (such as methods of inventory control). It also monitors drug utilization, focusing on high-cost drugs, and educates physicians about cost-effective prescribing patterns.

Utilization Management

Utilization controls are structured to be consistent with financial incentives and other organizational characteristics. *In general, HMOs have strong administrative controls on utilization or strong incentive programs, or both.* Some of the plans we studied believe that both are needed; however RIGHA and HCHP have few controls or incentives, relying instead on physician selection, ongoing education, and strong organizational culture to maintain efficient patterns of utilization. The range of utilization management mechanisms, many of which are used in combination, includes direct administrative controls, other incentives and deterrents (financial and nonfinancial), education and feedback for physicians, and peer review.

Direct Controls

Many HMOs impose procedural requirements with which providers and patients must comply. One of the most common is *prior authorization* for all elective inpatient admissions. Prior authorization may also be required for ambulatory services such as CAT (computerized axial tomography) scans, home health care, or costly drug therapies. Bay Pacific, Lifeguard, and Maxicare all require prior authorization for elective hospital admissions. HMO-PA requires notification but does not itself authorize admissions. Although it believes that preventing inappropriate admissions is crucial, it prefers to give physicians the incentive to hospitalize appropriately and avoid the role of granting or denying authorization.

Many HMOs will not authorize hospital admissions for procedures that can be performed on an outpatient basis. *Ambulatory* surgery *rules* tell providers what particular procedures and surgeries (for example, cataract removal or hemorrhoidectomy) the HMO expects to be performed in an outpatient setting unless special circumstances dictate otherwise. Both Lifeguard and HMO-PA have such a requirement.

Lifeguard will not authorize certain surgical procedures (for example, hysterectomies for women under age 35) without a *mandatory second opinion* from a consulting specialist that it selects. As part of its agreement with providers, some HMOs (Lifeguard, HMO-PA, Maxicare, Bay Pacific) specify that *pre-admission testing be performed on an outpatient basis or on the day of surgery.* Bay Pacific reports that 95 percent of its admissions are on the day of surgery. Lifeguard and HMO-PA have rules *prohibiting weekend admissions* in nonemergency situations.

The companion to prior authorization for hospitalization is inpatient *concurrent review,* which is conducted aggressively by some plans (Lifeguard, Bay Pacific, Maxicare) and less aggressively by others (HMO-PA, RIGHA, HCHP, SHARE, Capital Area). Still, every plan in the study devotes some resources to monitoring inpatient care. At Lifeguard and Bay Pacific, the status of every hospitalized member is reviewed daily by utilization review nurses, who talk by telephone with the hospital's nursing and discharge planning staffs. At Maxicare, length-of-stay estimates are reviewed at least every three days by utilization review nurses who do both on-site chart review and telephone monitoring. At other plans, only selected diagnoses are routinely monitored. For instance, HMO-PA focuses on patients who have been in the hospital beyond a reasonable time and on diagnoses that appear questionable or have the potential for alternative care, such as back pain.

Other Incentives and Deterrents

Other incentives and barriers may also affect both physician practice patterns and the care-seeking behavior of members. Except for the gatekeeper system, the incentives or barriers cited below have minimal effect in themselves and must be assessed in conjunction with other plan features.

A common way of controlling excess utilization is through the gatekeeper, or case manager, model, in which *a primary care physician must authorize all specialty referrals and hospital admissions.* Lifeguard, HMO-PA, SHARE, and Capital Area all use this approach. RIGHA has a modified gatekeeper system, in which members can refer themselves for selected specialty services (namely, dermatology, mental health, and gynecology). At HCHP, primary care physicians must authorize specialty referrals, but specialists may hospitalize patients without authorization from the primary care physician.

Some HMOs do not allow physicians extra time in their schedules for hospital rounds, creating an incentive not to hospitalize because *it is more convenient for physicians to see patients in the clinic.* Similarly, procedural barriers, such as having to complete a form, may deter physicians from making referrals in marginal cases. (HCHP, Bay Pacific, and HMO-PA require written referrals.) In addition, knowing that *referrals become part of their individual utilization profiles,* as at Lifeguard, may deter physicians, particularly if such profiles are used in performance evaluation.

HMOs have targeted copayments on specified services in order to control member demand for these services, avoid adverse selection, and keep premiums competitive. For example, copayments for mental health and emergency room services can be $20 per visit or more, although copayments for most visits are under $10. Some plans also *limit the number of ambulatory services* they will cover per year. For example, Lifeguard specifies that it will pay for only one complete physical annually, and virtually all plans limit the number of outpatient mental health visits. Finally, long waiting times for appointments with specialists, whether intentional or not, are another barrier.

The HMOs are increasingly providing members, and in some cases physicians, with *incentives for early discharge,* particularly for maternity care. For example, for normal delivery, HMO-PA gives mothers discharged within two days both a check for $75 and a home visit from a pediatric nurse practitioner. HCHP is testing programs to provide new mothers with home visits from homemaker aides and nurse practitioners. In addition, HMO-PA gives the obstetrician and pediatrician small payments for early discharge. It also pays physicians a case management fee of up to $300 per patient for supervising the delivery of home health services.

Finally, *many plans provide members with services not in the benefit package on a case-by-case basis when such services (such as a homemaker aide) could substitute for more expensive institutional care.*

Education and Feedback for and from Physicians

Communication with physicians has three main purposes:

— To inform physicians about the competitive environment faced by the plan

— To provide physicians with information about their own utilization patterns and about cost-saving alternative treatment modes

— To solicit physician input on all HMO matters (new programs to reduce utilization, ideas for improving service to members, tips on what the competition is doing, information on the type of contracting arrangements that hospitals seek, and so forth)

The last point is less immediately obvious, but most plans believe that it is critical. HMO-PA cited examples of how feedback from physicians has enabled it to improve its systems; for example, feedback resulted in the design of a better encounter form and in plastic membership cards for enrollees.

The plans approach communication differently. Maxicare has *quarterly dinner meetings* for participating physicians, with speakers on topics related to quality and utilization management; between 70 and 80 percent of medical groups are represented at least once each year. At RIGHA, all staff physicians and dentists belong to an association that meets frequently. Both SHARE and Capital Area have regular departmental and medical staff meetings. Maxicare and RIGHA have *pharmacy newsletters* with updates on generic drugs and cost-effective prescribing patterns (for example, when to treat acne with Accutane, a costly drug with potential side effects). Bay Pacific requires each new physician to attend an orientation meeting and publishes quarterly newsletters directed at IPA physicians.

The extent to which plans focus on the practice patterns of individual physicians varies, but many plans believe that such an emphasis is important in changing physician behavior. At HMO-PA, *practice statistics are provided* to each primary care physician office. Assistance on how to use and interpret the reports is also offered. Each month, primary care physicians receive data on their number of office visits, specialty referrals, hospital admissions, and hospital days per thousand members on their panel, all in comparison to the HMO-PA average. Physicians also receive lists of vendors with whom the plan has negotiated special rates for specific procedures (such as home care services).

Lifeguard has an impressive ability to identify physicians with inefficient utilization patterns through its automated ambulatory claims review system. The plan's feedback to physicians is mostly in the form of letters questioning a particular pattern of utilization. Participating physicians soon learn that the services they provide are incorporated into profiles against which the necessity of future services will be evaluated.

HCHP has traditionally evaluated utilization and performance at the health center level, although it intends to assess practice patterns of individual primary care physicians. Maxicare gives its groups in Southern California data on their utilization patterns each month. These reports, discussed by the medical group's utilization review committee, contain group-level data on hospital utilization and case- or physician-specific data when pertinent.

An HMO medical staff, physician group, or IPA may engage in regular *peer review*. This can involve medical record review, discussion of difficult cases, development of standards or protocols of care, and so on. At staff-model plans like HCHP and RIGHA, where opportunities exist for physician interaction and socialization, peer review is largely informal. Some medical groups—such as Maxicare's largest, the Hawthorne Community Medical Group—have established traditions of peer review that have been maintained in the HMO setting. In general, peer review, like quality assurance, tends to be more formal in an IPA, for logistical reasons. Lifeguard has successfully created a peer review system for widely dispersed physicians, many of whom are in solo or small group practice.

Quality Assurance

All plans articulate a concern for quality, although their endeavors assume various forms. Quality assurance is easier in staff-model plans because they have their own medical records, access to clinicians is easier, and physicians' salaries are reviewed and determined by the plan. Quality assurance in IPAs is more inspection-oriented, incurs higher costs (because physicians and records are decentralized), and may create greater resentment (because the intervention is more formal). Quality traditionally centers on clinical process and is largely assessed through retrospective review of medical records. Most HMOs have expanded their definition of quality assurance to include member access to care, which is typically measured in terms of waiting times for appointments. As described below, HCHP has broadened its view of quality to include many other aspects of health service delivery.

At RIGHA, under well-defined procedures for quality assessment, each department identifies its own areas of weakness through consultation with various staff members, including clinicians, consumer relations staff, and the medical director. Strategies for strengthening these areas are then formulated and approved by the board of directors. Lifeguard believes that quality of care is encouraged by emphasizing the physician-patient relationship and paying physicians on a fee-for-service basis, thereby avoiding incentives to underserve. Maxicare's quality assurance coordinators work with its physician groups in conducting medical care evaluations and other studies. They encourage these groups to adopt recognized professional standards (for example, Mayo Clinic standards for adult physicals and American Academy of Pediatrics standards for children) and then evaluate the groups accordingly, mostly through annual audits of charts. At SHARE, a quality assurance committee headed by a nurse practitioner examines complaints, periodic member surveys, and medical charts.

HMO-PA's attitude toward quality assurance is market-driven: it views a well-staffed, sophisticated consumer relations department as an ideal means for identifying problems in the delivery system. In addition to using the grievance process, consumers can highlight problems by changing physicians. The plan's annual process of recertifying physicians' offices includes surveys of member satisfaction as well as a review of telephone response time, number of grievances filed, physical appearance of offices, and practice statistics. A very large hospital or specialty referral bonus will generate a close examination of referral patterns to ensure appropriate use of consultants.

The approach HCHP takes is broader than the traditional approach. It views the quality audit function as analogous to that of the internal audit, and it reports directly to the plan's top management. The vice president for quality measurement is charged with developing quantifiable measures of performance, the equivalent of financial statements for financial performance. These measures include traditional health outcome indicators (such as perinatal complication rates) and measures of technical process (such as steps taken when a patient presents with acute chest pain). They also address access, which is defined as the ability to contact the plan easily by telephone, acceptable appointment and waiting room times, availability of after-hours and emergency care, and ease of referral to specialists. In the future, the plan hopes to assess continuity, coordination, and interpersonal elements of care. In its view, staff morale is important in assuring quality, as are characteristics of the physical environment, such as the privacy and dignity afforded patients.

Broadly, HCHP's goal is to establish norms of practice, by specialty or for a particular diagnosis, and then to reduce variance from those norms. Where there are clearcut standards of care, the plan attempts to monitor adherence to them. For example, its widely acclaimed automated medical records system notifies clinicians of patients who need follow-up care (for example, those who had abnormal results on a Pap smear) or who are at risk (for example, patients taking lithium carbonate or rubella-negative women who need immunization against German measles). Printed reminders are sent to clinicians to inform them that action has not been taken or that a checkup is due. However, HCHP has decided not to perform one traditional quality assurance effort—routine medical record or chart reviews—because it believes there are other, more direct methods of measuring and promoting quality.

Quality assurance and utilization control are closely related at most plans, although at HCHP the two functions are discrete. At Lifeguard, the same committee of physicians reviews both quality and utilization. At Maxicare, quality assurance nurses report to the director of utilization control, and the plan seeks to combine these two functions as much as possible. RIGHA's process is not formally linked to utilization control, but in many instances the problems addressed through the quality assurance process are related to utilization.

6

Corporate Philosophy and Management

Management can be conceptualized as entailing three functions. The first is leadership. This includes having a vision of the organization's future, creating a corporate culture, and communicating how each person's day-to-day activities contribute to the organization's mission. The second is actualizing that vision and culture in management decisions. The third is daily implementation, which includes attention to personnel issues, cash flow, administrative support systems, deadlines, data processing, public relations, and so forth. Lack of attention to, or improper execution of, these seemingly mundane functions is the downfall of many small, growth-oriented companies.

Overall Leadership

The HMOs in our study all exhibit a tangible, if at times difficult to describe, corporate culture. One important aspect is the belief that work is fun, a belief that is facilitated by rapid growth, which fosters opportunities for advancement and for the assumption of new and stimulating responsibilities. One way Maxicare maintains on-the-job excitement is by assigning to senior and middle managers projects that are outside their usual areas of expertise. This also helps develop a cadre of people who are knowledgeable across the plan. RIGHA seeks to create an environment in which employees feel responsible for each other's successes. It promotes the philosophy that nobody is expected to know everything, and therefore individuals should solicit help from others. Lifeguard also seeks to create an environment that encourages staff to seek help from each other.

Concern with quality of care is part of the culture at many plans. RIGHA and HCHP, both staff models, have gone to great lengths to instill the belief that, although costs matter, quality of care is primary. At Maxicare, an outside corporate director said that quality of care is the greatest concern of the board and is discussed at every meeting.

All of the plans exude a sense of optimism and energy. They believe that they are the best in the business, can overcome problems, and can adapt to changing environments. The drive to excel is strong. One executive at HCHP stated that the plan is "the most achievement-oriented organization I've ever known." Another commented that "every evening, half of the executive parking lot is full." RIGHA puts this attitude into operation in its careful selection of physicians, quality assurance programs, and reliance on teaching hospitals affiliated with Brown University. HCHP designs each new health center separately to avoid cookie cutter architecture, which might be more economical. HMO-PA has made major changes in its computer system virtually every year; systems staff are in close touch with top management and constantly strive to improve their products.

Leadership starts at the top, with the board of directors; however, *the role of the board varies significantly among the plans*, reflecting differences in plan origins, the personalities of board members and senior management, the distribution of ownership, and so forth. The board at RIGHA, for example, is instrumental in setting the tone of the organization and ensuring the accountability of top management, yet having a CEO whom the board respects has also proved to be important. The full board meets regularly and has four standing committees: finance and management, corporate planning, consumer relations, and professional relations. At the other end of the spectrum, the most important players on the board of HMO-PA and its parent corporation, U. S. Healthcare, are the plan's senior management; the outsiders on the board serve principally as advisors.

The directors of HCHP and SHARE act as sounding boards for long-term plans. The HCHP board includes several prominent individuals from the medical community and the community at large, thus enhancing the plan's image. The board approves budgets, capital expenditures in excess of $300,000, and all leases and major contracts. The SHARE board was instrumental in helping the plan raise capital for expansion.

The boards in several plans provide an outside perspective. Maxicare said that physicians on the boards of their individual plans articulate the provider perspective; also, serving on the board allows physicians to participate in policymaking. At the corporate level, one board member, an executive with Universal Studios who has no formal background in health care, has been a business confidant of the CEO for many years. At Lifeguard, the director of personnel and compensation at Hewlett-Packard, a large electronics firm, provides assistance on personnel, management, and long-range planning issues and reflects the attitudes of a large employer.

Another important aspect of leadership is the personality and abilities of the chief executive officer. Two traits stand out. The first is entrepreneurial drive. As we discussed in chapter 3, many of the plans were the first in their communities, and the spirit of innovation persists today. Maxicare, SHARE, and U. S. Healthcare (the parent company of HMO-PA) are all multistate organizations and are expanding rapidly. Maxicare has also created a national accounts program as part of its effort to become accepted nationally. The program enables an employer to sign a single contract for coverage at multiple locations, obtain identical benefits, and receive a single bill. Chapter 4 presents other examples of entrepreneurship, for example how SHARE set out to attract Medicare and other nongroup enrollees, how SHARE and Maxicare were the first in their communities to be federally qualified and to avail themselves of the federal mandate, and how all of the plans have sought to expand their provider networks.

The second trait is the longevity of both the CEO and much of the management team. Maxicare, HMO-PA, Lifeguard, Bay Pacific, Capital Area, and SHARE are still run by their founders, and many of the senior managers have been with the plan from its inception or shortly thereafter. This reflects both an exciting work environment and opportunity for advancement. Many businesses falter as they grow because the innovative skills necessary at the start are different from the skills required to manage a large organization. Clearly, the leaders of the plans in our study have met that challenge.

Strategic Management

All of the HMOs can be characterized as having *an ability to integrate the various functions*, such as marketing, finance, provider relations, and claims processing, and also display what Fred Wasserman, chairman of Maxicare, describes as "organizational balance." Achieving organizational balance has been critical in light of the growth that the plans have experienced. Examples of organizational balance include

— Designing the utilization review system to focus on problems that might be created by the financial incentives that the physicians face

— Assuring that delivery capacity is expanding rapidly enough to meet the demands created by enrollment growth

— Not losing sight of quality considerations in the drive to reduce costs

— Carefully planning which functions to centralize and which to decentralize

— Adjusting management styles and practices as the number of employees grows

All of the HMOs have had to decide how much to centralize the various functions of the plans, particularly the multistate corporations that oversee several plans. The tendency of several of these corporations has been to centralize. Maxicare, a multistate company, processes claims and maintains its enrollment and billing files at a single location; sets all of its rates from the corporate headquarters; and exerts strong corporate supervision over the marketing function. Plan marketing directors (with the exception of the California director) report to the marketing director for the corporation rather than to the executive director of the individual plan. This centralization facilitates control over the plans during a time of rapid expansion, relieves the individual plan executive directors of the burden of having to hire and supervise people with certain technical skills (such as data processing and actuarial skills), and maintains a consistent product from the employers' and consumers' perspectives. At the same time, most HMOs allow considerable autonomy in the delivery of medical services, preferring to rely either on financial incentives (SHARE, Maxicare, HMO-PA) or on a shared value structure (RIGHA, HCHP).

Another characteristic is *strong systems of internal communication*, which promote both coordination in day-to-day decision making and shared values. Maxicare makes extensive use of electronic mail, which the chairman feels not only speeds and enhances communication but also allows the organization to function with fewer layers. Maxicare and HMO-PA have created systems to assure that consumer grievances are communicated to top management. HMO-PA avoids detailed job descriptions and fosters the attitude, especially among senior management, that anyone on the staff is available to help anyone else. Lifeguard and RIGHA promote the view that there is no such thing as a dumb question, thereby encouraging staff who face new situations to approach others for help. RIGHA has frequent staff meetings and retreats, which from a narrow, efficiency-oriented perspective might seem superfluous. (Maxicare, on the other hand, minimizes the number of formal meetings.) All of the plans espouse participative management, although styles differ among the plans, and some are more hierarchical than others.

Ease of communication also facilitates *an ability to act quickly in response to both marketplace opportunities and internal threats*. For example, Maxicare and SHARE were the first HMOs to use the federal dual-choice mandate in their respective communities; Maxicare submitted its request for qualification even before the application forms were designed. One executive at Maxicare commented that, by the time most organizations had finished planning, Maxicare had already taken action.

Management Execution

The day-to-day aspects of management receive scant attention in either business or popular literature. Best-selling books are written about different corporate and leadership styles, and corporate intrigue is the topic of numerous novels and television shows. To our knowledge, nobody has produced even a third-rate soap opera about such matters as personnel development, accounts receivables management, the investment of cash assets, or the updating of computer systems. Yet when these functions are not performed properly, the resulting drama can be riveting.

Many of the plans *invest heavily in training programs*, most of which are developed internally. Those for marketing representatives were described in Chapter 4. Both HMO-PA and Maxicare have extensive training programs for member services (consumer affairs) representatives. Maxicare, for example, devotes two weeks to classroom and one week to on-the-job training. HMO-PA also has a program to train provider relations staff. HCHP sends physician managers to executive training courses at top business schools. In addition, several of the plans, including SHARE, HCHP, Bay Pacific, and Capital Area, regularly hold management retreats, in part as a training device.

The plans also pay *close attention to financial management*, assuring that bills are rendered on time and that cash reserves are immediately invested, mostly in safe short-term instruments. The plans have different philosophies on speed of claims payment. At one extreme, Lifeguard seeks to process most clean claims (that is, those that are complete and do not raise any utilization or other questions) within a few days in order to maintain good relations with physicians. Another plan was delaying payment by six weeks at the time of our study, but only because its growth had exceeded its computer capacity; it was working to achieve a three- to four-week payment cycle.

One problem that has plagued many plans which have found themselves in financial difficulty is incurred but not reported claims, that is, claims for services that a provider has rendered but for which a bill has yet to be submitted. All of the plans feel that they have good control over such claims. Costs of services that are authorized in advance can be estimated with some accuracy, and patterns are analyzed to estimate other incurred but not reported claims.

All of the plans pay *attention to data-processing and information systems*. Maxicare has created a separate computer system and software development subsidiary. All Maxicare executives have computer terminals on their desks; the corporation has more than 900 terminals, of which some 600 are in Southern California for use by the local plan and by the corporate offices. Lifeguard is able to process most claims within 48 hours, and staying current on data entry is viewed as the key to effective ambulatory utilization review, at which it excels. HMO-PA has developed a comprehensive approach to information systems. It starts with a list of employers for marketing representatives to contact. Once an employer agrees to offer the plan, the prospects file is transformed into the group and enrollment file for purposes of billing, issuing enrollment cards, handling enrollee inquiries, statistical analyses, and so forth. The data files are carefully designed so that each relates to the others. In cooperation with an outside vendor, RIGHA has developed software packages for managing staff-model HMOs; it is considering marketing these software packages to other plans.

7

Conclusion

Some persons have suggested, only partly in jest, that managing an HMO that would at least break even used to be easy. Only a few simple practices had to be followed. First, utilization review or reimbursement incentives needed to be sufficiently effective that hospital use was kept 20 to 30 percent lower than that in fee-for-service plans, not a difficult task in most communities. Second, adequate controls were needed over incurred but not reported claims. Third, common sense had to be exercised in marketing (until recently, there were likely to be only one or two other HMOs in the community, so one could use the Title XIII dual-choice requirements to gain access to employees and obtain sufficient enrollees to break even). Fourth, good relations with physicians were important, not a big challenge once the physicians realized that the HMO had a positive effect on their incomes and work hours.

This list might be supplemented with a few other guidelines that could be followed by anyone who has decent management instincts, reasonable interpersonal skills, and an understanding of health services delivery and financing. Indeed, one of the CEOs with whom we met wisecracked that, in the current growth environment, his plan's success did not require great talent.

Actually, managing an HMO is not easy. Sharper skills are required today than even five years ago because of the veritable revolution taking place in health care financing and delivery. By the same token, even sharper skills are likely to be needed in the future. Although HMO growth is rapid and shows no signs of abating, individual HMO marketplaces are becoming more crowded, and some of the competitors are not likely to survive. As an illustration, until about two years ago, New Orleans was the last city of its size not to have an HMO; today, at least six HMOs are competing with one another. The Chicago area, hardly a hotbed of activity until recently, now has more than 20 HMOs in various stages of development or operation, and numerous PPOs are being formed. Several of the HMOs we visited for this study report competition from new entrants to the market. In one case, competition forced a plan to keep annual premium increases considerably below past levels.

Employers and insurance carriers are increasingly placing restraints on the fee-for-service system, thereby reducing the utilization differentials that HMOs can achieve. In doing so, they are emulating the approaches that HMOs have originated and refined. Primary among these is utilization review, which has sparked the emergence of firms that perform preadmission and concurrent review nationally by telephone. Indemnity carriers and employers are also beginning to negotiate prices with hospitals and other providers. They are taking steps to shift the locus of care from inpatient to ambulatory settings. Finally, some large corporations, such as Owens-Illinois in Toledo and Zenith in Chicago, have created patient advisory services to steer employees to efficient providers. Although the impact of these cost management efforts has not been systematically studied, some dramatic results have been reported. For example, some large corporations report that reductions in rates of inpatient utilization by indemnity plan enrollees have exceeded 30 percent in some locations.[1]

Our study is a snapshot of a small sample of highly successful HMOs at a particular time. One can only speculate on how the findings might differ if this study were repeated in a few years. Nonetheless, we can distill some central characteristics that are likely to contribute to success in a less forgiving environment.

Superior management will become even more important. The plans that thrive will have leaders who are innovative and capable of rapidly turning threats into opportunities. They will also be able to integrate the various functions of the plan, for example synchronizing the utilization control mechanisms with the financial incentives, assuring that delivery capacity is expanded consistent with enrollment growth, and not losing sight of quality of care in the interests of constraining costs.

Related to the traits of flexibility and creativity is the need to stay abreast of a marketplace that is rapidly changing. This entails both redesigning products and adding to the range of products. Some HMOs are responding to the threat of PPO growth by using the HMO's provider network and cost management skills to develop their own PPO, thereby appealing to the consumer's desire for a broader choice of providers. Staying in touch with the marketplace also requires an ability to differentiate the plan from competing plans, effective communication programs with employers and prospective enrollees, and a skillfully designed and professionally conducted sales effort. It will also entail marketing to new populations, notably Medicare enrollees, small businesses, and, in some states, Medicaid beneficiaries.

The successful plans will respond to the needs of employers and enrollees. Employers are increasingly demanding data on performance and greater flexibility in HMOs' premium-setting practices. The HMOs may also have to be more flexible in tailoring benefit packages.

Having satisfied enrollees is a prerequisite to continued growth. Successful plans will find ways of cementing consumer loyalties and differentiating themselves from the competition so that they are not competing only on the basis of price. One way of building loyalty is to have an accessible network of providers who are consumer-oriented and who offer high-quality care. Staff- and group-model (closed-panel) HMOs in particular will need to contract with fee-for-service providers to improve accessibility. The plans will have mechanisms for identifying employee problems early, dealing with them promptly, and taking steps to reduce reoccurrences.

Finally, good relations with physicians, particularly those who deliver primary care, are essential, especially in situations where most participating physicians contract with several plans and can urge patients to shift from one to another. Furthermore, with the proliferation of HMOs, physicians will increasingly shop around among HMOs and be more selective in their contractual arrangements. Fostering good relationships requires good communication, reimbursement mechanisms and amounts that are perceived as fair, assistance in patient management (such as by advising on good office management practices and by making available comparative data on utilization patterns), a balance between the need for adequate utilization controls and the avoidance of paperwork and procedural burdens, and recognition of the physician's desire for clinical independence.

An HMO has three principal stakeholders: the enrollees, the physicians, and the plan itself, as represented by the owners or board members and the employees. An impressive feature of all of the plans we visited was their attitude that all three must gain from the relationship. This attitude, along with their talented and energetic managers and staffs, will stand them in good stead in future years.

Note

1. A. Webber and W.G. Goldbeck, "Utilization Review," in Peter D. Fox, Willis G. Goldbeck, and Jacob J. Spies, *Health Care Cost Management: Private Sector Initiatives* (Ann Arbor: Health Administration Press, 1984), pp. 69–90.

Part II
Maxicare California

8

Introduction

Maxicare California is a federally qualified, investor-owned, network-model HMO. It is the original and largest plan operated by Maxicare Health Plans, Inc. (MHP). Headquarters of MHP and Maxicare California are in Los Angeles. This case study focuses primarily on the California region, particularly the Southern California service area.* Selected activities of the corporation as a whole are also discussed when relevant to the California plan.

Maxicare began operations in 1973 with a Medicaid contract from the state of California. It formed a partnership with the 10 physicians in the Hawthorne Community Medical Group at that time and was incorporated as a nonprofit health plan. Today, MHP is a for-profit, publicly traded corporation with more than 700,000 members in 13 states at the time of our site visit. (With the acquisition of HealthAmerica and HealthCare USA, the national membership exceeded 2 million at the end of 1986. Based on total enrollment, MHP is the largest investor-owned HMO chain in the United States. Maxicare California is still the largest plan, with 245,000 enrollees as of June 1985 (see table 8.1) and 1,400 physician members.

In Southern California, Maxicare contracts with more than 30 medical groups, most of which are multispecialty, for all physician services. Groups are financially responsible for any referral

---

*Maxicare California as a legal entity includes the company's activities in Northern as well as Southern California. Maxicare has few members in Northern California, and its operations there were not examined for this study.

Table 8.1

Maxicare Membership Growth

Year*	Members All Regions	California	Increase in California (%)
1974	2,845	2,845	
1975	3,909	3,909	37
1976	6,252	6,252	60
1977	18,563	18,563	197
1978	25,249	25,249	36
1979	58,363	58,363	131
1980	87,631	87,631	50
1981	187,996	117,278	34
1982	227,390	143,056	22
1983	288,274	161,022	13
1984	460,412	208,753	30
1985†	600,670	245,242	17

* As of December.
† As of June.

care not available within the group and are responsible for negotiating fees. Maxicare is at risk for hospital care; however, targets are set and surpluses are shared equally between Maxicare and the medical group that generated them. The medical group is not at risk for hospital overruns.

Despite increasing competition, MHP has maintained an impressive enrollment growth and a strong balance sheet. This is due in part to its ability to innovate and adapt. MHP was one of the first HMO chains to establish a program to market to national employers. It has a Medicare program—Maxicare 65—in Los Angeles and Chicago, and a major new hospital capitation program is underway in Southern California. In addition, several of the newer health plans involve joint ventures with local physician groups, reflecting the corporation's view that ownership has a positive impact on success and quality of care.

In addition to the various health plans, MHP owns six pharmacies (all in Southern California), a hospital (jointly with other investors), HCS Computer, Inc. (a computer service company), and HealthCare Alternatives, Inc. (which conducts utilization review for private employers).

Financial performance is notable. Premium revenues of MHP reached $304.9 million in 1984, compared to $113.5 million in 1982. In the first quarter of 1985, they were $107.6 million, equivalent to an annual rate of $430.2 million, an almost fourfold increase in three years. Net income before taxes also increased dramatically, from $2,507,000 in 1982 to an annualized rate of $14,848,000 in 1985 (based on first-quarter performance), a sixfold increase. The company is widely recommended by investment analysts as both a good short-run and a good long-run investment. To quote William Blair and Company, "Since 1981, when it converted to a for-profit corporation, it has experienced annual growth of 60 percent in membership, 73 percent in revenues, and 150 percent in earnings. We expect the company will reach its goal of 1 million members and $1 billion in revenues no later than 1988, two years ahead of schedule."[1]

This report is an account of some of the reasons for the success of Maxicare. Chapter 9 characterizes the medical marketplace in which the plan operates. Chapter 10 presents an overview of the plan and addresses such topics as the plan's history, relationships to physicians and hospitals, quality assurance and utilization review, marketing, consumer relations, and corporate philosophy and business operations. Finally, the factors that appear to account for the plan's success are summarized in chapter 11.

Note

1. William Blair and Company, *Basic Report 85–15*, 25 February 1985, p. 1.

9

The Market

The demographic and economic characteristics of Maxicare's service area are favorable for HMO development. The population of Southern California is growing, well educated, and slightly more affluent than the U.S. population as a whole. However, the medical market is disciplined and highly competitive, and the area is characterized by low hospital utilization and relatively efficient practice patterns, creating a more difficult environment for rapid HMO expansion.

This chapter presents data for the counties in the service area of Maxicare's Southern California plan and compares them to national averages.

Demographic and Economic Characteristics

Maxicare serves seven counties surrounding greater Los Angeles. Its service area stretches along the coast from Santa Barbara to San Diego and extends east to the desert as far as Palm Springs.

The total population of these seven counties exceeds 13.6 million, of which more than half resides in Los Angeles County (see table 9.1). That county's population grew by about 6 percent between 1970 and 1980, compared to 13 percent for Santa Barbara County and more than 30 percent for the other five counties. The comparable figure for the United States as a whole is 11 percent.

The service area population is generally younger than the national average, slightly more affluent, and better educated (see table 9.1). In only two counties, representing less than 10 percent

Table 9.1

Population and Socioeconomic Characteristics of Maxicare's Southern California Service Area

County	1980 Population	Change Since 1970 (%)	Median Family Income, 1979 ($)	Over Age 65, 1983 (%)	Below Poverty Level, 1979 (%)	Unemployment Rate March, 1985 (%)	High School Graduates, 1983 (%)
Los Angeles	7,477,503	+ 6.2	21,125	9.9	13.4	6.5	69.8
Orange	1,932,709	+36.0	25,918	8.3	7.3	3.8	80.4
Riverside	663,166	+45.1	18,681	14.9	11.3	8.1	68.9
San Bernardino	895,016	+31.2	20,038	10.0	11.1	7.0	71.0
San Diego	1,861,846	+37.1	20,304	10.3	11.3	5.5	78.0
Santa Barbara	298,694	+13.0	21,630	11.3	10.6	6.3	79.1
Ventura	529,174	+39.8	23,602	8.3	8.0	6.6	75.9
Total	13,658,108						
U.S. Average		+11.4	19,917	11.7	12.4	7.1	66.5

Source: U.S. Department of Commerce, Bureau of the Census, *County and City Data Book—1983* (Washington, D.C.: Government Printing Office, 1983); U.S. Department of Labor, Bureau of Labor Statistics, personal communication.

of the service area population, are 11 percent or more of the residents over age 65; the national average is between 11 and 12 percent. In only one county (Riverside) is the median family income below the national average of $19,900. The highest incomes are in Orange County ($26,000 median); Los Angeles County's median family income is $21,000. The percentage of the population living below the poverty level is less than the national average in all counties except Los Angeles; there it is 13.4 percent, compared to the national average of 12.4 percent. Unemployment rates vary but are generally lower than the national rates. All seven counties are above average in terms of the population's education.

Medical Cost and Supply Factors

The medical market in California is disciplined, probably due to its long experience with prepayment in general and the Kaiser Permanente Health Care Programs in particular. Utilization rates on the West Coast have traditionally been among the lowest in the nation. Utilization data are striking: by every measure, the counties in Maxicare's service area are below national norms for hospital utilization (see table 9.2). For example:

— Admissions per thousand persons in the population in 1983 ranged from 103 in Ventura to 136 in Los Angeles, compared to 159 for the United States as a whole.

— Average length of stay varied from 5.2 in Ventura to 6.9 in Los Angeles, versus 7.6 nationwide.

— Reflecting the low admission rates and length of stay, inpatient days per thousand persons in 1983 ranged from 535 in Ventura to 933 in Los Angeles, compared to 1,206 nationwide.

— Hospital occupancy rates in 1983 ranged from 62 percent in Orange to 69 percent in Riverside–San Bernardino, compared to the national average of 74 percent.

Supply of hospital beds is also low, ranging from 2.3 per thousand persons in Ventura County to 3.9 in Los Angeles County, which is below the U.S. average of 4.5. Even San Diego, a teaching center, has only 2.8 beds per thousand persons. On the other hand, most of these counties have higher physician-to-population ratios than in the U.S. average of 2.1. Santa Barbara has the highest ratio, with 2.8 physicians per thousand persons; Los Angeles has 2.7, and San Diego has 2.6.

Table 9.2

Medical Cost, Utilization, and Supply Factors in Maxicare's Southern California Service Area, 1983

County	M.D.'s per 1,000 Persons	Inpatient Days per 1,000 Persons	Admissions per 1,000 Persons	Hospital Beds per 1,000 Persons	Average Length of Stay (Days)	Occupancy Rate (%)	Hospital Expenses per Capita ($)
Los Angeles	2.7	933	136	3.9	6.9	66	649
Orange	2.5	715	121	3.2	5.9	62	526
Riverside and San Bernardino*	1.9	769	124	3.1	6.2	69	473
San Diego	2.6	684	105	2.8	6.5	67	427
Santa Barbara	2.8	775	125	3.3	6.2	64	423
Ventura	1.8	535	103	2.3	5.2	63	311
United States†	2.1	1,206	159	4.5	7.6	74	560

Source: American Hospital Association, *Hospital Statistics* (Chicago: AHA, 1984); American Medical Association, personal communication; U.S. Department of Commerce, Bureau of the Census, *Statistical Abstract of the United States, 1985* (Washington, D.C.: Government Printing Office, 1984).

* Only combined data are available.

† Data for the U.S. metropolitan statistical areas, except for M.D.'s per 1,000, which represents the overall U.S. average.

Although utilization rates in Maxicare's Southern California service area are low, hospital expenses per capita in Los Angeles County are some 15 percent higher than the U.S. average. Although fewer units of service are consumed, the cost per unit is higher, creating above average total costs. In the service area, hospital expenses per capita range from $311 in Ventura to $649 in Los Angeles, compared with a U.S. average of $560. Los Angeles is the only county in the service area with above average hospital costs.

The Health Insurance Market

The health insurance market in this service area is highly competitive, with HMOs vying against each other as well as against indemnity plans, as the relatively high HMO enrollment suggests. Maxicare's major competitors are Health Net, Pacificare, CIGNA, Kaiser, Family Health Plan, and other plans in specific parts of the service area (see table 9.3). There are 14 HMOs besides Maxicare in Southern California; about 25 percent of the population belongs to an HMO (including Maxicare).

Other competitors include Blue Cross and Blue Shield, commercial carriers, hospital chains offering both prepaid and indemnity plans, and PPOs. Maxicare is concerned about competition from plans with flexible and more limited benefit packages, such as those offered by Humana Care Plus, but believes it is well positioned to compete, especially with the advent of Project Window (described in chapter 10). When asked about the impact of PPOs on Maxicare's business, the president and chief operating officer, Pamela Anderson, said she views them as "creating IPAs for us." The marketing director said that this year PPOs started to have an observable impact on Maxicare; however, most Maxicare executives do not believe that PPOs pose a long-term threat.

Table 9.3

HMOs in Maxicare's Southern California Service Area

Plan	Year Formed	Model	Members, December 1984
Maxicare Health Plans, Inc. Hawthorne	1973	Network	207,000
Kaiser Permanente of Southern California Los Angeles	1945	Group	1,773,300
CIGNA Healthplan Glendale	1929	Group	373,600
Health Net Van Nuys	1979	Network	308,000
FHP, Inc. Fountain Valley	1961	Staff	101,900
Pacificare Cypress	1978	Network	95,000
General Medical Centers Anaheim	1972	IPA	84,600
Greater San Diego Health Plan San Diego	1980	IPA	72,900
United Health Plan (Watts Health Foundation) Los Angeles	1973	Network	57,300
Inland Health Plan San Bernardino	1981	IPA	30,400
Protective Health Providers San Diego	1979	Group	26,000
Health Group International Los Angeles	1982	IPA	14,000
Serra Health Plan Sun Valley	1972	Group	13,000
Inter Valley Health Plan Pomona	1979	IPA	12,800
VIP Health Plan Oxnard	1982	IPA	8,700

Source: Modification from InterStudy, *National HMO Census* (Excelsior, Minn.: InterStudy, 1984).

10

Overview

Maxicare's leaders have demonstrated a talent for capitalizing on opportunities (see table 10.1).[1] The HMO Act was passed during Maxicare's first year of operation, and in 1976, when the plan was eager to expand its membership, it became the first federally qualified HMO in California. Even before the federal law had been fully implemented, while employers were still unfamiliar with its meaning and the industry unsure of employer reaction, Maxicare used the mandate to gain access to a large number of major employers that continue to form the core of its Southern California business. Another transition came two years later, when Maxicare moved away from the single-group model and began to contract with medical groups other than the Hawthorne Community Medical Group in Southern California. At the same time, it assisted the Hawthorne group in expanding its sites.

In the late 1970s, Maxicare's leaders recognized that, to obtain the capital necessary for continued growth, conversion to for-profit status would be advantageous. At the end of 1980, Maxicare became the first California HMO to convert to a for-profit corporation. In the restructuring that accompanied the conversion, MHP, a for-profit holding company, was created, and Maxicare California became a wholly owned subsidiary. MHP also acquired various other entities affiliated with the HMO, including three pharmacies, a computer service company, and a building partnership.

Another opportunity spotted and acted upon by management was the purchase of the old Fox Hills Hospital, now Maxicare

Table 10.1

Significant Dates in Maxicare's History

Date	Event
August 1972	Maxicare was incorporated as a nonprofit corporation.
February 1973	Maxicare became operational.
March 1976	Federal qualification was obtained.
March 1977	Rapid growth in enrollment began.
January 1978	Maxicare contracted with other medical groups in Southern California to expand delivery sites.
December 1980	Maxicare became a for-profit corporation; Maxicare Health Plans (MHP), a for-profit holding company, was created.
August 1981	Fox Hills Hospital (now Maxicare Medical Center) was purchased.
December 1981	Fremont General acquired a 94% interest in MHP.
June 1982	MHP expanded out of California by buying all outstanding shares of CNA Health Plans (HMOs in Illinois, Indiana, and Wisconsin), now Maxicare Midwest Health Plans.
January 1983	Maxicare Texas (Houston) became operational.
January 1984	Maxicare Missouri (St. Louis), Maxicare Utah (Salt Lake City, Provo, and Ogden), and Maxicare Northern California (San Francisco) became operational.
September 1984	Maxicare 65, a Medicare risk contract, became operational in Illinois.
January 1985	Maxicare Louisiana (New Orleans) and Maxicare Ohio (Cincinnati and northern Kentucky) became operational; Maxicare North Texas (Dallas) formed through partial purchase of North Texas MedCare.
February 1985	Fremont General sold its remaining 55% of shares of MHP common stock through a public offering.
July 1985	Maxicare 65 opened enrollment in California.
August 1985	Exclusive contract with Hawthorne Community Medical Group expired; Maxicare Arkansas (Fort Smith) became operational.
September 1985	Project Window became operational.
January 1986 (Projected)	Maxicare–UHS Nevada (Las Vegas and Reno) became operational; Maxicare Arizona (Phoenix) became operational.

Medical Center, from Humana, Inc. in 1981 for $4.5 million. The hospital was bought in partnership with physicians in the Hawthorne group and other investors (MHP owns 51 percent) and is in an area with a heavy concentration of Maxicare members. MHP provides the administrator and other support personnel, while physicians from the Hawthorne group staff the hospital.

In 1981 and 1982, Fremont General acquired a 94 percent interest in MHP, mostly by purchasing shares held by founding physicians in the Hawthorne group. As part of this arrangement, Fremont General obtained four of seven seats on the board of directors, although day-to-day management remained in the founders' hands. In retrospect, top management believes MHP benefited from this move, which shifted control away from physicians and created a strong financial base.

The next milestone was Maxicare's expansion out of state. In mid-1982, Maxicare purchased the HMOs in Illinois, Indiana, and Wisconsin owned by CNA Insurance. Maxicare management agreed to Fremont General's terms regarding the sale—namely, that if the new venture lost more than $1 million, MHP would sell it. This entity became Maxicare Midwest; it has grown from 70,000 members at the time of acquisition to 245,000 members today. At that point, MHP had to learn how to run a national company. This involved deciding which functions to centralize and which to handle locally. The company's basic philosophy, which has not changed, was to centralize as much as possible.

Since 1982, MHP has expanded at the rate of one or more new regions per year (see table 10.2). The company tends to focus on major markets (for example, Chicago, Dallas–Fort Worth, St. Louis, New Orleans, Cincinnati, Salt Lake City, Houston, Las Vegas). It is also starting up in smaller markets, however, some of which are near its hub cities (for example, Fort Smith, Arkansas). Many of the newer health plans are joint ventures between MHP and local physician groups. Maxicare believes such arrangements facilitate expansion, because local ownership provides motivation and enhances physician relations.

The plan entered into a Medicare risk contract, effective July 1, 1985, following the successful experience of the Illinois plan. Several adjustments are being made to reflect the unique characteristics of this population. The new program, known as Maxicare 65, places greater emphasis on in-home services, including high-tech services such as infusion therapy and enteral and parenteral nutrition. Although the lock-in is stressed in communications

Table 10.2

Maxicare Health Plans, September 1985

Plan	Status of Subsidiary*
Maxicare California	Wholly owned
Maxicare Midwest	Wholly owned
Maxicare Texas	Joint venture with Kelsey-Seybold Clinic, P.A. (67% owned)
Maxicare Missouri	Joint venture with South Grand Health Services, Inc. (80% owned)
Maxicare Utah	Joint venture with Salt Lake City Clinic (89% owned)
Maxicare Louisiana	Joint venture with Browne-McHardy Clinic (80% owned)
Maxicare Ohio-Kentucky	Wholly owned
Maxicare North Texas	Joint venture with First Texas Medical, Inc. (67% owned)
Maxicare Arkansas	Joint venture with Holt-Krock Clinic, Inc. (87% owned)
Maxicare–UHS Nevada	Joint venture with Universal Health Services (50% owned)
Maxicare Arizona	Wholly owned (to become operational January 1986)

* In several cases, the partner in a joint venture has been granted an option to buy additional shares up to a negotiated percentage.

with Medicare enrollees, it will be enforced leniently at first because some misunderstanding is viewed as inevitable. The approach to marketing has also been adapted to the Medicare population. These efforts will rely in part on community meetings in churches, senior citizen centers, health care facilities, and so forth.

The company continues to innovate, as it believes it must. Two new programs, discussed later in this chapter, are the national accounts program to accommodate employers with multiple locations and Project Window, a plan for capitating hospitals and their medical staffs.

The medical groups are the focus of Maxicare's delivery system. Maxicare evolved from a group model with a single large group practice to its present network arrangement by contracting with additional multispecialty physician groups. The plan's usual practice is to contract with the hospitals already used by the group and with a conveniently located pharmacy, creating a local delivery unit. In Southern California, the plan contracts with more than 30 physician group practices (comprising about 1,400 physicians in over 80 locations) and over 50 hospitals. A significant portion of inpatient days is at Maxicare's own hospital. Maxicare has different arrangements (usually IPAs) in some of its other regions and has departed from its basic network model in Southern California by capitating hospitals, as described in Project Window.

Members gain access to the delivery system by choosing a medical group location (all family members must enroll in one medical group). Next, they are encouraged to select a primary care or family physician (internist, family practitioner, pediatrician, or, in some groups, obstetrician-gynecologist). Maxicare's brochure lists medical group locations, together with the associated pharmacy and hospital or hospitals, so that in choosing a medical group, members are aware of the other providers they are electing. In addition, some medical groups have their own after-hours or urgent care clinic. Enrollment literature informs new members that they are only covered for physician and hospital services rendered or referred by their primary care physician.

Maxicare offers its employer groups two core benefit packages plus a series of optional, supplemental riders. The two benefit packages differ in price and in cost sharing by patients. For example, the copayment for most office visits is $2 in the higher priced "basic" plan and $10 in the less expensive "preferred" plan (see table 10.3). The preferred plan also has a copayment of $300 per hospital admission. Both plans cover most ambulatory services and provide unlimited acute-care hospitalization. Diagnosis and treatment for alcohol and drug abuse are covered on an inpatient or outpatient basis, as medically appropriate, but rehabilitation services are excluded. Emergency care is covered both in and out of Maxicare's service area. Extended care, home health, and ambulance services are covered, as are health education, medical social services, and family planning.

A variety of supplemental benefits, some with different levels of cost sharing, can be purchased by the employer to supplement either the basic or the preferred plan. These include

— Detoxification and rehabilitation for drug and alcohol abuse at no charge

— Refractions for persons of all ages (persons under age 18 covered in basic and preferred)

Table 10.3

Maxicare California Benefit Options

Service	Preferred Copay ($)	Basic Copay ($)
Physician office visits	10	2
Physician home visits	10	5
Health assessment (under age 18, includes vision, hearing, and developmental testing; unclothed physical; laboratory work; immunizations; and dental screening)	25	2
Periodic checkups (including laboratory and X ray)	25	2
Laboratory tests, X rays, cytology	—	—
Surgical operations (outpatient or hospital)	—	—
Hospital care	300 per admission	—
Emergency visits (hospital or office of non-Maxicare physician)	50% of charges (50 maximum)	50% of charges (25 maximum)
Alcohol and drug abuse (diagnosis and detoxification only)	50% of charges	50% of charges
Outpatient mental health services	10 first visit 30 thereafter, up to 20 visits per year	20 first visit 20 thereafter, up to 20 visits per year
Home health services	10 per visit	—
Physical therapy (outpatient)	10 per visit	2 per visit

Table 10.3—continued
Maxicare California Benefit Options

Service	Preferred Copay ($)	Basic Copay ($)
Therapeutic injections, inoculations, and immunizations	10 if visit is for injection only	2 if visit is for injection only
Family planning		
IUD insertion	25 (does not include device)	25
Vasectomy	75	50
Tubal ligation (elective)	200 (includes hospital cost)	100
Abortion (elective)	200 (includes hospital cost)	185
Fertility counseling and testing	50% of hospital and physician charges	—
Diaphragm fitting	25 (does not include device)	—

— Eyeglasses
— Inpatient psychiatric care
  14 days covered or
  45 days covered
— No charge for office visits
— No charge for family planning services
— Durable medical equipment
— Option of expanding 20-visit mental health benefits by
  covering more than 20 visits with $10 copays or
  waiving copay for first 20 visits or
  both
— Dental benefit (low and high options)
— Prescription drugs ($2, $1, and zero copay)

Excluded from all Maxicare coverage are psychiatric conditions which, in the opinion of the utilization review committee, are not subject to improvement by short-term therapy; cosmetic surgery for no medical reason; custodial care; extensive long-term neuromuscular rehabilitation; sex change operations; oral surgery for orthodontic purposes; experimental procedures; and treatment of temporal mandibular joint syndrome unless due to specified medical conditions.

Relations with Providers

Maxicare's provider network offers broad geographic coverage and extensive choice among physicians. In Southern California, more than 30 medical groups in 80 locations and 50 hospitals, as well as about 40 pharmacies, are affiliated with Maxicare. Medical groups are the starting point, and Maxicare has excelled at helping physicians organize their practices to treat HMO patients in a cost-effective manner without imposing overly rigid systems or formulas upon them. In this section we first describe Maxicare Southern California's relations with physicians, then relations with hospitals and other components of the provider network, and finally a new contracting scheme known as Project Window.

Physicians

The largest medical group in Southern California is still the Hawthorne Community Medical Group. It has about 160 physicians and serves nearly half the Maxicare members in Southern California (about 120,000 persons). The other 30 or so physician groups serve the remaining half; the smallest of them may have only two or three physicians and perhaps 300 enrollees. Many groups are also members of other open-panel HMOs. On the average, prepayment accounts for between 40 and 50 percent of the patient revenues of Maxicare's physician groups in Southern California; in contrast, the Hawthorne group is about 80 percent prepaid, and most of its HMO patients are Maxicare members.

The relationship with the Hawthorne Community Medical Group is a special one, built on history and tradition. Overall relations are good, although certain ties have been severed over the last few years. Originally, it was agreed that Maxicare would not use other physician groups in areas that the Hawthorne group already served or would like to begin serving and that the Hawthorne group would not contract to provide services for any competitor of Maxicare. Operationally, this meant that Maxicare gave the Hawthorne group the option to expand into any area of Southern California where Maxicare wanted a physician group, which lowered Maxicare's growth. As of August 1985, however, both Maxicare and the Hawthorne group can freely contract with others, and both have already taken steps to do so. (The Hawthorne group, for example, has signed contracts with Aetna Choice and Health Net.) The Hawthorne group will continue to staff Maxicare Medical Center and be compensated for doing so.

Signing up new physician groups has not been a problem; Maxicare reports that medical groups tend to approach the HMO rather than vice versa. Maxicare seeks high-quality groups that are located near employee homes and that have excellent reputations in the community. Contracts are signed with new medical groups mostly because a new site would be helpful in marketing to particular employers or because there is a hole in the plan's geographic coverage.

In California, an average of three medical group applications is received each week, but fewer than 1 in 10 is seriously reviewed. Only one medical group in California has lost its Maxicare contract as a consequence of providing inferior care, a situation the HMO tries to avoid by careful screening. Pamela Anderson reviews every application before a contract is signed.

Prospective medical groups must complete an application, undergo a site visit, and pass a quality assurance audit. The application collects information on the licensure, specialties, board status, hospital privileges, and office hours for each physician in the group. It requires documentation of malpractice insurance and an explanation of the group's procedures for handling matters such as after-hours calls and referrals to specialists. Financial statements are requested to ensure that groups are well capitalized and fiscally sound. Resumes are submitted for both physicians and the group's administrators. Information on the physical plant is also collected in the application, including total square footage and number of examining rooms.

During the site visit, a member of Maxicare's provider relations staff conducts a thorough study of the office, including its operations and environs. The facilities are surveyed for adequate parking, access (for example, elevators), physical appearance, cleanliness, signs, and so forth. Maxicare asks about the group's relations with hospitals, and the pharmacy, if there is one, is studied for location and hours of operation. The report that is prepared includes a characterization of the community, and data are collected on patient mix, for example, the proportion of Medicare and Medicaid patients. The administrator is interviewed to assess his or her knowledge of prepayment, and the information systems are reviewed. Finally, Maxicare obtains a sample of patient names and contacts patients to solicit their views of the medical group.

The third component of the precontract review is another site visit, this time by a registered nurse from the quality assurance program. Charts are sampled—10 each from pediatrics, medicine, and obstetrics-gynecology—to assess standards of care. Record-keeping practices are examined to see if charts are well organized, separated by dividers, and so on. The facility is checked for the presence of a crash cart, for the safekeeping of drugs, and for the availability of staff certified in cardiopulmonary resuscitation (CPR). Waiting times for urgent, routine, and full physical appointments are reviewed.

Once the group is accepted, a contract is entered into. The terms vary to some extent by group. All groups are capitated, but the level of capitation will vary, depending on the services that are included. Maxicare always assumes the risk for hospital care, home health care, and out-of-area coverage. The medical group is always at risk for primary care, most specialty care, and ancillary services. However, some groups receive a lower capitation in exchange for Maxicare's assuming the risk for particular procedures or types of care, such as nuclear scans, pediatric neurosurgery, or other highly specialized services.

New Maxicare medical groups must appoint a medical director, decide which physicians will be considered primary care providers, establish an internal compensation scheme, and set up utilization control and quality assurance processes (discussed below). Maxicare proffers guidelines and recommendations to groups but rarely dictates policy.

Methods of physician compensation within medical groups vary depending on group preferences and traditions. Although Maxicare advocates capitation, and in fact capitates primary care physicians and specialists in other locations, most groups in Southern California operate on a fee-for-service basis. Thus, individual physicians are generally paid on the basis of productivity, with a percentage of fees withheld to cover any overruns beyond the capitation received from Maxicare.

Maxicare does not restrict out-of-group referrals, which, particularly in smaller groups, may be necessary. Groups can make arrangements with whomever they wish for specialty care; however, the groups are at risk for most specialty care up to a predetermined stop-loss per patient per contract year. Medical groups negotiate their own rates with specialists, and many report that, to keep Kaiser at bay, subspecialists accept fees below their usual charges, often as much as 35 to 45 percent below.

Although physicians and medical groups are not at risk for hospital care, Maxicare shares hospital budget surpluses with them. To the extent that a group is under its hospital budget, Maxicare and the group split the surplus equally.

Hospitals and Other Providers

Hospitals, pharmacies, and other ancillary providers complete the delivery system. Maxicare owns (jointly with the Hawthorne group) Maxicare Medical Center, a hospital in Culver City, and it also contracts with more than 50 community hospitals. In addition, the plan will begin in September 1985 to capitate 15 prestigious hospitals in Los Angeles to provide the full range of physician and hospital services.

Maxicare Medical Center is licensed for 103 beds and currently operates 76. It is used predominantly by three medical group locations with a total enrollment of about 70,000. Although most persons admitted to the hospital are Maxicare members, the hospital does allow United Health Plan, another HMO, to admit some patients (most of them obstetric). The hospital was renovated after its purchase in 1981. According to hospital administrator Tom Avery, MHP chairman and chief executive officer Fred Wasserman's instructions to him were to "make it look like a hotel." One popular feature is an attractive birthing room, which indeed has the amenities and decor of a hotel. The hospital handles about 150 deliveries per month and has a neonatal intensive care unit. It does not have an emergency room, nor does it perform neurosurgery or open-heart surgery. The three operating rooms averaged nearly 1,200 procedures each in 1984, a high proportion of them outpatient surgeries. Maxicare is currently contemplating a major project to further renovate, expand, and modernize the facility, with an estimated price tag of $16 million.

Maxicare's relations with other hospitals have traditionally reflected the preferences of its medical groups. Typically, Maxicare approaches the hospital that a medical group wishes to use, provided that the hospital meets Maxicare's standards for quality, reputation, and location. The plan views the reputation of the hospital as important in marketing, and many of the participating hospitals have teaching programs. In negotiations with the hospital, Maxicare does not guarantee a particular volume of patients; consequently, the plan usually finds it easier to achieve favorable rates over time, as hospitals recognize the importance of Maxicare's business to them. If a high-cost hospital is reluctant to negotiate, then Maxicare may not be able to accommodate physician preferences. In the vast majority of cases, however, either the hospital and Maxicare come to terms, or the physician group realizes that a more efficient hospital will best serve the group's interests by increasing the opportunities for generating savings, in which the group shares.

The mechanisms for paying hospitals vary. They can be negotiated per diems, flat discounts off usual charges, or a per case rate similar to a diagnosis-related group (DRG). Maxicare rarely pays full per diem charges, except for services such as inpatient detoxification or normal delivery, where the length of stay can be predicted and controlled. Overall, Maxicare prefers to purchase hospital care on either a per diem or discounted fee-for-service basis. The plan does not care whether the rate is a per diem or a discount, since it is easy to calculate what each means in terms of the other. Maxicare's negotiated per diems average at least 20 percent off usual charges.

   Hospital rates may vary by patient volume and promptness of payment. For example, Maxicare may be guaranteed at least a 10 percent discount at a hospital, but that discount could go as high as 20 to 24 percent if volume is high. In other cases, Maxicare may pay one per diem rate for the first three days of maternity care and a lower rate thereafter. Maternity rates may include pediatric care for newborns as well. With regard to speed of payment, the agreement may entail a discount of 15 percent for claims paid within 30 days, 12 percent for those paid within 45 days, and 8 percent for payments received after 45 days.

   Maxicare owns one inpatient and six outpatient pharmacies and contracts with between 30 and 40 retail pharmacies. The plan has no direct contracts with surgicenters. It is in the process of reevaluating its home health care contracts and may choose to use a more limited number of vendors in the future. It also has contracts with dental providers, optometrists, physical therapists, and other specialized providers.

Project Window

Project Window was conceived by Fred Wasserman and so named because it represents a window of opportunity for the HMO. In a departure from its usual practice, Maxicare has enlisted 15 high-quality high-profile hospitals—many of which are teaching institutions—and their medical staffs. The plan believes that these high-utilizing physicians affiliated with prestigious hospitals are interested in Maxicare for one main reason—the erosion of their practices due to growing enrollment in managed delivery systems. Maxicare is willing to contract with them because the plan is able to fully lay off risk to the physicians and hospital. The physicians, who will belong to a hospital-based IPA, and the hospital will each receive 39 percent of monthly premium revenues. The HMO will keep the remaining 22 percent to cover marketing, administration, and emergency and out-of-area care. Professional services are automatically reinsured after a stop-loss of $5,000 per patient per illness. Hospitals can purchase reinsurance from Maxicare if they choose.

   The new hospital capitation is expected to have impacts at many different levels. It is likely to attract members who have not elected HMO coverage in the past. These patients will now have more access to top hospitals, a wider selection of physicians, and easier access to specialists of their choice than other HMOs offer.

Wasserman feels this will enable Maxicare to compete more effectively against the new plans offered by proprietary hospital chains, such as Humana Care Plus. In addition to benefiting the patient, Maxicare is no longer at risk for hospital services and thus can reduce its close monitoring of hospital utilization. Maxicare intends to stay involved to the extent that physicians and hospitals not accustomed to tracking and controlling utilization may need and request assistance. The hospitals stand to benefit from increased volume; their combined average occupancy rate dropped from about 76 percent in 1980 to 68 percent in 1984.

Project Window is a logical step in two ways. First, it is consistent with Maxicare's belief in the importance of a broad and complete delivery system—the project will add 1,300 physicians and 15 hospitals to Maxicare's network. Second, Maxicare has increasingly sought to have providers assume risk—and the new venture passes financial risk for hospital services to the participating hospitals. This is not an unmitigated blessing, however: Maxicare cannot absolve itself of all responsibility, since it does not want the project to fail; and, by decreasing its own risk, Maxicare also decreases its potential gain. An open question is the effect the new program will have on enrollment in Maxicare's medical groups, since some crossover is likely.

Utilization Control and Quality Assurance

An explicit goal of the plan is to combine utilization control and quality assurance as much as possible. Indeed, one department houses both functions, and the staff responsible for quality assurance report to the director of utilization control. The structure is somewhat in flux, because the department is reorganizing and adapting to the new requirements of Project Window and Maxicare 65 (the program for Medicare enrollees).

Utilization Control

Responsibilities for utilization control are shared between the medical groups and the plan. Maxicare in Southern California has nine utilization control coordinators (all registered nurses), an authorization supervisor, and three authorization clerks. These staff work with the medical groups on utilization control issues, with assistance from the regional medical director as needed.

In general, each medical group forms a utilization review committee of four to seven physicians, with assistance from a Maxicare utilization control coordinator. The committee typically meets weekly. The company believes utilization review should be the responsibility of a committee exercising peer review, not of one or two physicians making decisions. Maxicare suggests that primary care physicians be well represented on the committee and that physicians rotate through the committee so that a broad cross-section of medical group members is exposed to the process. There are usually representatives from internal medicine, family practice, pediatrics, obstetrics-gynecology, and surgery; sometimes psychiatry is represented. Some groups compensate physicians for this service, while others do not. The committee is actively involved in both prior authorization and retrospective review; concurrent review is handled for the most part by the Maxicare utilization control coordinators.

All medical groups are urged to institute prior authorization for expenses that are paid for through the group's capitation, although they are not required to and a few groups in California do not. (All expenses for which Maxicare is at risk, such as hospital and home care services, must be authorized in advance by Maxicare. Groups have an interest in controlling these expenses as well, because they share equally in hospital budget surpluses.) Each group determines what must receive authorization, but a fairly typical list would include

— Treatment to last two or more weeks (for example, physical therapy)
— Speech therapy
— Laboratory tests not frequently ordered or not performed on-site (for example, genetic testing)
— Amniocentesis
— Hospital admissions, particularly surgical (urgent cases by a utilization control nurse over the telephone, semi-urgent by group medical director, elective by committee)
— Referral to specialists, in or out of the medical group
— Psychiatric care, inpatient and outpatient, including developmental testing
— Laboratory, radiology, or other procedures totaling more than $200
— Plastic surgery referrals

— Alcohol and drug abuse referrals

— Corrective appliances in excess of $300

Maxicare has developed a list of surgical procedures that can usually be performed in an outpatient setting. Further, groups are required to perform preadmission testing in an ambulatory setting whenever possible.

In reviewing authorization requests, the committee acts as a gatekeeper. It receives a copy of the patient's chart, consultation reports, results of laboratory tests, and any other pertinent information. While perhaps 90 percent of all requests are approved, committees can and do defer decisions until more information is received or deny permission altogether. Every committee has a list of specialists to whom it can refer particular problems or questions. Committee decisions are recorded on the authorization forms, and copies are sent to Maxicare.

All contracted providers (hospitals, home health agencies, and so on) are aware that an authorization number is required for payment from Maxicare. Hospital admitting offices typically call Maxicare, at which time an authorization clerk verifies that prior approval from the medical group has been obtained. The clerk also checks eligibility and benefit coverage, issues an authorization number, and sets a preliminary length of stay based on the 50th percentile of the Professional Activity Study (PAS) guidelines.

The concurrent review process is triggered as soon as an authorization number is issued. At this time, a Maxicare utilization control coordinator becomes responsible for reviewing the admission within one working day. Concurrent review generally takes place on-site, with most hospitals allowing access to patient charts, but it may be conducted by telephone. Maxicare coordinators have no contact with patients, but they do interact with hospital discharge planners and physicians. Maxicare believes that one weakness of its concurrent review program is the absence of any review of ancillary services: the focus is almost exclusively on length of stay. The coordinator uses both screening criteria developed by Maxicare and the InterQual Intensity of Service, Severity of Illness, and Discharge Screens (ISD) standards to determine the appropriateness of the admission and revise the PAS length of stay. Additional reviews are conducted at least every three days until the time of discharge.

Automated hospital utilization monitoring reports, updated daily, provide the utilization review staff with current information on hospitalized patients. The reports contain information on each patient, including the medical group, hospital, admitting physician, length of stay, diagnosis, and type of coverage. A new information system is currently being developed.

Retrospective review is also encouraged by Maxicare. The Maxicare coordinator assigned to the medical group regularly assembles utilization data, both general and case- or physician-specific. As Maxicare sees it, retrospective review has both a utilization control and a quality assurance function. Maxicare suggests retrospective review of the following:

— Overall inpatient days per thousand members, admissions per thousand, and trends in average length of stay

— Number of admissions and nature of diagnosis per physician (to identify overutilization and inappropriate admissions)

— Average cost per inpatient day (to identify increases in hospital rates and overutilization of ancillary services)

— A sample of hospital bills (for educational purposes)

— Number and type of outpatient referrals, laboratory tests, and X rays ordered per physician (to identify over- and underutilization of services)

— Use of Relative Value Scale code by physicians within a specialty (similar services should have similar charges)

— Inappropriate hospital admissions

— Inappropriate approvals for emergency room visits

— Access surveys

— Quality assurance audits

The success of Maxicare's utilization review efforts is measured principally in terms of hospital days per thousand members. Maxicare's current target in Southern California is 350 days per thousand for the non-Medicare members.

Quality Assurance

Maxicare requires that each medical group establish an internal quality assurance program. This usually takes the form of a committee, which may or may not be the same committee that conducts utilization control. Minutes from the meetings and all recommendations must be submitted quarterly to Maxicare's regional medical director. It is also recommended that minutes be disseminated to all medical group physicians.

Quality assurance committees at the medical group level review grievances, analyze the findings of Maxicare's annual audit (described below), review retrospective utilization data, and initiate discussions of other issues affecting quality of care and member access.

Maxicare in Southern California has two quality assurance coordinators, both of them registered nurses, who work with the groups and are responsible for

— *Precontract medical group reviews* (as described in the section on provider relations)
— *Yearly on-site audits* to review medical charting standards and both adult and pediatric standards of care (90 charts per medical group facility are reviewed each year)
— *Member access surveys* (formerly handled by the consumer affairs department)
— *Technical assistance* to medical groups as needed for data collection or other quality-related projects

The on-site audits consume a large proportion of the quality assurance coordinators' time. These are essentially spot checks on charting practices (for example, whether results of laboratory tests have been read and signed off on by physicians) and on adherence to pediatric and adult standards of care. Each group is judged on the basis of its own stated standards of care. For example, Maxicare suggests that the Mayo Clinic frequency standards be followed for adult screening, but groups may choose to follow other standards or to develop their own. For pediatric care, Maxicare suggests the American Academy of Pediatrics' guidelines. In addition, the American Cancer society's guidelines have been adopted for cancer screening.

In all quality assurance endeavors, the regional (Southern California) medical director acts as a resource for the nurses, for individual physicians, and for the medical directors of the physician groups.

Marketing

As the first federally qualified HMO in California, Maxicare relied heavily in its early days on the federal mandate in marketing. The plan reports that it was also conscientious in delivering on promises and was willing to create new satellite physician offices to match the locations of large employers in Southern California. Because the plan has now signed up most large employers within its service area and acceptance of HMOs is widespread, the federal mandate is believed to be of little value. Indeed, many large employers offer more than the two HMOs that the federal law requires.

Aerospace companies have from the start been a mainstay of Maxicare, representing four of the five largest accounts in Southern California (Hughes Aircraft, Northrup Aviation, Rockwell International, and Garrett Corporation). The fifth is the Los Angeles Unified School District. No single firm represents more than 1 percent of total enrollment.

In addition to the plan's California focus, the corporation as a whole has a national accounts program to market to and service multistate employers. This program enables a large employer to sign a single contract for coverage at multiple locations, obtain identical benefits, and receive a single bill. The premiums charged are those set for each Maxicare plan and vary by location. Some 400 corporations participate in this program, and Maxicare reports that it has contracts with more Fortune 500 companies than any other HMO in the United States.

Some 80 percent of new enrollment is from increased recruitment within existing employer groups. Marketing efforts are heavily oriented in this direction and toward enrolling new medium-sized employer groups and Taft-Hartley trust funds. The plan does not accept groups with fewer than 25 employees, nor does it enroll persons who are not group members (except for Medicare beneficiaries and conversions when enrollees leave employment).

One key to Maxicare's marketing success is the service it provides employers and members. The plan seeks to sign up physician group practices that deliver high-quality care and takes great pride in its consumer affairs department, which is available to solve individuals' problems. In addition, postsale service to employers is emphasized. Service standards require that a marketing representative visit a large account at least six times a year; a medium-sized account, four times; and a small account, twice. An effort is made to spot problems and find ways to provide ongoing service, not just service at contract renewal time. The plan is also willing to be flexible. As described above, it can tailor benefits more than most HMOs and will open new facilities to meet the needs of employers. For example, Maxicare contracted with a medical group in Palmdale, which is some distance from Los Angeles, because the community had a significant number of Rockwell International employees.

Another key to success is proper hiring. The staff of the Southern California plan consists of a marketing director, some 10 marketing representatives, four service representatives, and clerical support. The service representatives fill entry-level positions and are commonly promoted to marketing representative. Marketing representatives should be "enthusiastic, smart, and career-oriented." All of the Southern California staff are women with prior sales experience, all are college graduates, and some have teaching credentials. The plan seeks marketing representatives who care about what they sell and demonstrate integrity. Their compensation is mostly in the form of salary, in order to avoid incentives to oversell. Bonuses are paid twice a year. They average only 20 percent of salary, although in rare instances they have exceeded 100 percent.

The plan has a carefully designed training program, which is conducted by the corporate office for all Maxicare plans. It includes presentations by speakers from the major departments, discussions on how to listen to employers and build rapport with them, and instruction on how to explain the Maxicare product, including how utilization review, second opinions before surgery, and so forth contribute to the quality of care. All marketing representatives rehearse the presentations they will make to employers. The presentations are standardized, partly for legal reasons, to assure that the same message is delivered at all of the plans. Prospective representatives are expected to become conversant with the contents of a lengthy training manual, and there are daily quizzes.

Once in the field, marketing representatives are assigned geographic territories. They have quotas; for example, they must make 12 personal visits a week, of which five are initial presentations and seven are follow-up or service calls. The sales message stresses the quality of care provided, including the importance of the peer and utilization review functions and the role of the con-

sumer affairs department. Other plan features that are emphasized include

— Coverage that, unlike the typical indemnity plan, is easy
  to understand
— Low out-of-pocket payments
— Breadth of the provider network, which facilitates access
  to services
— Health education programs

Once an employer has agreed to offer the plan, the marketing representative helps implement the offering. The representative may, for example, prepare notices for the company news-
paper as well as draft and reproduce a letter for the employer to
send to employees. Maxicare offers free wellness programs at the
workplace for all employees, not just those who enroll in the
plan. These programs include smoking cessation, weight control,
and stress management.

Marketing is supported by extensive advertising, particularly
on television. The advertising budget amounts to roughly 1 percent of total premiums. Advertisements do not mention the term
"HMO," in order to avoid generic advertising for HMOs; instead,
they stress the positive features of Maxicare.

The marketing department has also taken steps to facilitate
communication between the individual marketing representative
(and, hence, the employers) and Maxicare's top management. All
representatives report directly to the plan's marketing director. In
addition, they are free to talk individually with anyone in senior
management and to bring problems to their attention. For example, a marketing representative reported that Hughes Helicopter
was unhappy with the plan's substance abuse programs, and
corrective action was taken. Representatives record all sales contacts, including telephone calls, on computer, and these reports
are available to top management. A computerized data base allows the national director to find out the status of any employer
group contacted by Maxicare, including when it was last contacted, by whom, whether it offers Maxicare, and, if so, the number of employees enrolled.

The plan credits its marketing success largely to the quality
of the product and customer service. This success is noteworthy
because Maxicare's premiums tend to be above those of other
plans, including other HMOs. Furthermore, many of the physician

groups to the south and east of Los Angeles are also providers for Health Net, the Blue Cross HMO. In many instances, employers offer both plans (and employees have access to many of the same physicians), yet Maxicare has been a highly successful competitor.

Consumer Affairs

The consumer affairs department believes that the better educated members are and the better service they receive, the better Maxicare's retention rate will be. The main functions of the department are to

— Reassure members and educate them about Maxicare's services and benefits

— Resolve claims issues and problems, including management of the grievance process

— Act as liaison between providers and members

Most complaints relate to quality of care, claims denied (usually out-of-plan), and access (waiting times in clinic). The department also performs special services for members when possible, such as making appointments for them and helping them change physicians. There are about 32 consumer affairs representatives in Southern California, four supervisors, four regional managers, and a director. In addition, a national consumer affairs office at the corporate level serves all MHP regions.

Consumer affairs representatives are required to have a college degree. Beyond that, the director looks for decision-making ability. Representatives from all regions are trained together in a formal, three-week program developed by the national consumer affairs office. The first week is primarily an orientation to the plan's various departments; the second focuses on understanding the procedures manual; the third consists of on-the-job training, which includes monitoring calls to ensure that wrong information is not conveyed.

One representative is hired for every 6,000 to 8,000 members. The expected workload is 30 calls per day and 10 grievances per month, although the calls increase during open enrollment periods. The plan receives 1,000 or more incoming calls each day, resulting in an average of 200 to 250 grievances per month; this number is used as a barometer of the service the plan is providing. About 2 percent of all *calls* are medical, while about 30 percent of all *grievances* are medical. Of these, only one or two per month turn out to be serious problems.

About a dozen representatives are assigned to the central office, while the other 20 are in the field on either a full-time or rotating basis to serve individual medical facilities. The plan believes that if members can walk into a consumer affairs office while they are upset, problems can be addressed before they fester and enrollees will not convey negative impressions of the plan at work or at home. Another public relations plus is the fact that representatives have the power to authorize payment of claims up to $100. The director believes this helps the morale of both member and representative when legitimate claims merit it. However, this authority is used only for clear cut cases, not cases that require research.

When a telephone or walk-in complaint is received, a representative records the information on a grievance form. A second form is used to itemize the problem, the extent and type of research needed, and the deadline for responding. An acknowledgement letter is sent to the member, thanking him or her for calling, promising an answer within 30 days, and providing a form that the patient may fill out to express the problem in his or her own words, if desired. The complaint is then investigated. If patients feel they were not treated appropriately or on a timely basis, for example, extensive research is carried out. The representative will get a statement from the patient, from the physician, and from the medical director of the group or facility. If it is an issue of quality of care, then all medical records and test results are examined. A specialist's opinion may be solicited. All of this is presented to the regional (Southern California) or corporate (MHP) medical director, who will make a decision. Within the allotted time period, a response is sent to the member. The last paragraph of the letter always informs members of the next step they should take if not satisfied with the results. In this event, they can request a hearing, which will be held within 15 days of the request. Such dispute hearings occur every month or two; all concerned parties attend, the executive director of Maxicare (Southern California) acts as arbitrator, and the member receives a letter from MHP's president within 30 days giving the resolution.

Consumer affairs representatives use the computer in two main ways. First, they have access to member accounting information to determine eligibility and to check coverage provisions.

Second, a computerized grievance filing system, known as GRIPE, has been developed to track complaints by department (X-ray, pharmacy, and so on), by medical group, by employer group, and by nature of the complaint (for example, medical staff, policies, access). This enables the department to identify trends in order to spot problems early.

The director of the department submits a weekly report to the regional executive director (Southern California) and to the national consumer affairs office. The report contains

- Number of calls received, by type
- Number of calls per thousand members
- Number of walk-in complaints
- Number of calls from new advertising (for example, Medicare promotion)
- Narrative of trends
- List of the most important cases, including all cases with risk management implications (including possible malpractice or other litigation, significant cost to the corporation, and adverse publicity)

Corporate Philosophy and Business Operations

Fred Wasserman attributes the organization's success in part to dramatic changes in the market during the late 1970s and early 1980s that were conducive to HMO growth. However, it was the business philosophy and the way which that philosophy was put into operation that allowed the plan to capitalize on favorable changes in the environment. In this section we discuss selected aspects of the corporate philosophy, the role of the board at both the corporate and the plan level, the role of computer systems, and rate setting and financial management.

Corporate Philosophy

Wasserman and others articulate the following principles as characterizing Maxicare

- Flexibility and a focus on opportunity: For example, Maxicare purchased CNA Health Plans for $7.5 million, or 1.5 times book value, as its initial expansion outside of

California. At that time (1982), CNA had 70,000 enrollees; the plans that were part of CNA now have 200,000 members.[2]

— Orientation toward the market and customers: Maxicare is willing to tailor benefit packages and to sign contracts with new medical groups, even in remote areas, to meet employer needs. In addition, Maxicare is seeking to create "brand health care" through its national marketing program, which already serves some 400 multistate (mostly Fortune 500) corporations.

— Emphasis on training in public health: A large proportion of the senior management (including the president and executive vice president) has graduate degrees in public health. Such training is viewed as conducive to understanding the delivery system and the mind-set of providers. It may also explain why Maxicare spends more per member on health education than other HMOs.

— Strong management and team spirit: Managers are characterized by high energy, an ability to act quickly, good team spirit, and the view that work is fun. Turnover is low, and corporate headquarters has not lost any senior staff in the last two years. One problem, however, is a shortage of executive directors, although two to three persons are being trained for these positions each year through an informal program.

— Delegation of authority: There are few layers of management. The president, for example, has 10 to 12 people who report directly to her. Most management staff are not allowed to become overly specialized and may be assigned tasks or special projects outside their normal areas of responsibility to help them grow professionally and to encourage versatility.

— Use of computer systems: Reliance on the computer for day-to-day planning, tracking, and communication permits the organization to function more informally (which may appear paradoxical) and with fewer layers. Computer systems are discussed in greater detail later.

— Demand for excellence: The CEO believes the organization generates peer pressure for good performance and successfully minimizes corporate politics. Each member of the senior executive staff is capable of running a plan and thus is respected in the field for his or her knowledge of operations.

— Ability to make decisions quickly: This characteristic flows from the open communication and absence of a bureaucratic structure. One person commented, "We never have formal meetings."

Maxicare has a seven-year strategic plan; however, Pamela Anderson commented that serious planning was realistic only for a one- to two-year period. Another executive commented that the strategic plan was less important than the ability to think strategically. He expressed the view that, in the time most organizations take to develop a plan for a new undertaking, Maxicare would have implemented it.

Concomitant with the informality is considerable centralization. Claims processing, rate setting, premium collection, and accounting are all performed at corporate headquarters. The corporate office oversees the marketing function, including most advertising decisions. Even expense reports are reviewed by the president of the corporation as well as the regional executive director. We were told that feedback on routine matters was prompt and was facilitated by the electronic mail system.

Maxicare has national offices of program evaluation (responsible for utilization control and quality assurance), consumer affairs, and provider relations that develop MHP policy and coordinate its implementation across regions. The national directors have no line authority over health plan staff, who report instead to their own executive directors. National directors do play a major role in hiring and training new staff for the regions, as well as in providing support to regional staff and ensuring some consistency of approach in these functional areas throughout the organization. The national marketing director plays a slightly different role, working with large employers to coordinate their accounts across regions.

Role of the Board

Boards exist at both the corporate and the plan level. The MHP board has seven members, of whom three are insiders (management) and four are outsiders. It meets quarterly. One outside board member said that quality of care was the board's greatest concern and that it was discussed at every meeting. He felt that the corporation should accept a lower return on the shareholder's investment, if necessary, to assure quality and that doing so was in the corporation's long-term financial interest.

Board members regularly receive financial reports, budgets, expansion plans, utilization reports, and so forth. A major emphasis of the discussions is on strategic decisions, such as expansion and the development of new products.

The board for the Southern California plan has nine members, three from corporate management (including the chief executive officer and the chief operating officer), three physicians, and three consumers. Nonmanagement members are paid for serving. The board sets strategies and reviews grievances, marketing plans, and financial performance. Although ultimate authority resides with corporate headquarters, the board gives providers and others at the local level a sense of participation and a vehicle for contributing to decision making.

Computer Systems

Maxicare has established its computer staff as a wholly owned but legally separate corporation—HCS Computers. That corporation receives from Maxicare 57 cents per member per month for its services. Having a separate subsidiary that receives payments based on a fixed charge allows Maxicare to budget better, creates an incentive for the computer staff to provide the most comprehensive service within a fixed budget, and reflects the different values and compensation structure of computer system staff compared with health plan staff.

Overall, Maxicare is highly automated. There are about 950 terminals nationwide, of which 650 are in Southern California (for both corporate headquarters and the plan). Most executives have terminals on their desks. The computer staff develop and maintain all software, except that for the accounting function. This includes the software necessary for determining eligibility, tracking marketing efforts, reviewing utilization, billing, and processing claims.

Because computers are regarded as an important tool for senior management, the computer systems' staff meet regularly with management. This helps managers understand the capacity of computers and their application to various business functions. Maxicare has grown into a large computer purchaser and can negotiate favorable arrangements with vendors.

Table 10.4
Monthly Premium History for Maxicare California,
January 1975–1985*

| Year | Monthly Premium ($) | | |
	One Party ($)	Two Parties ($)	Three Parties ($)
1975	23.99	47.98	73.82
1976	33.34	66.68	99.60
1977	37.78	75.73	108.85
1978	42.18	82.37	119.85
1979	42.18	82.37	119.85
1980	47.91	98.95	141.23
1981	53.00	107.00	159.04
1982	63.70	130.10	193.10
1983	77.74	158.73	235.59
1984	85.09	173.64	258.17
1985	91.94	187.74	279.00

* Between 1975 and 1979, premiums were revised each January. Starting April 1979, they were revised at various times during the year. The table presents the monthly premiums in effect in January of the year listed.

Rate Setting and Financial Management

The plan uses strict community rating but is considering adopting more refined rating structures. Strict community rating is viewed as having several advantages. First, it facilitates budgeting. Second, breaking the enrollee population into cells, each with its own rate, would introduce instability into the premiums paid by individual employee groups due to random fluctuations. One person commented, only slightly tongue-in-cheek, that "we are not sophisticated enough" to adopt a complicated rating structure (implying that there are advantages to avoiding unnecessary complexity).

Table 10.4 shows Maxicare's premium history for the last 10 years. Rates are developed largely by projecting current experience rather than through independent actuarial estimates. In the past, premiums were driven largely by medical care costs, but they are becoming increasingly constrained by competition. Nonetheless, recent increases are significant, even if below past levels. Between January 1981 and January 1983, annual increases have averaged just below 22 percent, whereas they were 9.5 and 8.1 percent, respectively, in the subsequent two years. One result of both the size of the plan and the heightened pressure to restrain premium increases is that Maxicare is becoming more aggressive in negotiating hospital rates.

The plan has tight administrative controls. Expenses, such as travel vouchers, must be approved at senior levels. Annually, each manager prepares a budget for his or her department showing staffing, salary totals, and other costs. However, budgeting is difficult in an era of rapid growth. The plan has also negotiated favorable long-term leases and contracts for photocopying services, and generally seeks to be a prudent buyer.

Notes

1. For a more detailed history of Maxicare, see Touche Ross & Co., *Investor's Guide to Health Maintenance Organizations*, DHHS publication no. (PHS) 82-50185 (Washington, D.C.: Government Printing Office, 1982), pp. 83–89.

2. The price at the time of purchase corresponded to $107 per member; in contrast, transaction prices are now around $500 per member, although this has varied considerably.

11

Success Factors

While the reasons for Maxicare's success are accurately described by Fred Wasserman (chapter 10), three factors are particularly noteworthy. These are Maxicare's talent for seeking and capitalizing on business opportunities, its customer orientation, and its organizational balance. The first two are from Wasserman's list; the third is an amalgam. It is, however, a term that Wasserman used himself 10 years ago to characterize the successful HMOs he studied for his doctoral dissertation.[1]

Focus on Opportunity

Several examples of Maxicare's capacity for spotting and seizing opportunity have been discussed in this case study. The most obvious include the decision to become federally qualified (Maxicare submitted its request for qualification before the Department of Health, Education and Welfare had even developed an application form); the acquisition of its own hospital; the expansion into the Midwest with the purchase of CNA; the development of a national accounts program; and the capitation of hospitals and their staffs on a large scale to expand rapidly the provider network in Southern California. In addition, Maxicare was the first California HMO to convert to for-profit status when a state law was passed allowing HMOs to do so. It was also the first HMO in California to advertise extensively on television. While in some cases Maxicare's timing has been fortuitous, the company's list of firsts is too long to attribute to luck alone.

Orientation Toward Customers

Maxicare's strong marketing program, its attention to postsale service, and its preoccupation with consumer relations all contribute to a definite customer orientation. Maxicare markets service rather than price, and it delivers. For example, the company assists employers with offerings, provides free health education programs to all employees (not just enrollees), has on occasion created new sites to meet employer needs, and offers a flexible benefit package structure that includes a high and low option, numerous supplemental riders, and a Medicare program. In addition, consumer affairs representatives are available on-site in many of the larger medical groups, an unusually large investment in member relations. Finally, Maxicare has created a win-win situation with its physician groups, maximizing the probability that members will be well served. The plan recognizes that physician attitude and behavior are not under management control, and when an HMO's relations with physicians are strained, customer service may suffer.

Organizational Balance

One aspect of organizational balance is the integration of functions. In comparing successful and failed HMOs in his doctoral dissertation, Wasserman concluded that lack of organizational balance may explain failures. He wrote:

> In examining the effects of decision making which is directed toward one particular aspect of the organization, it becomes apparent that consideration is infrequently given to the effect of the decision on the other parts or sub-systems of the firm. For example, the decision to increase enrollment without considering physician staffing may produce consumer dissatisfaction and deterioration in the quality of care.

Health maintenance organizations must integrate the delivery of health services with sound business practices. While the elements of organizational balance are difficult to pinpoint, some examples from Maxicare may illustrate its presence there:

— Financial accountability of providers without incentives strong enough to jeopardize quality of care

— Strategic thinking and planning, yet quick decision making

— For-profit organization, with heavy representation of public health school graduates among senior management

— National offices to coordinate functions across regions, with local staff reporting along traditional lines to executive directors of individual health plans

— Emphasis on service at reasonably competitive prices

— High expectations of staff, with commensurate rewards

— Experimentation with new lines of business, while maintaining strong growth in core business

— Standardization and centralization combined with flexibility and responsiveness to local concerns

Note

1. Fred W. Wasserman, "Health Maintenance Organizations: Determinants of Failure or Success," doctoral dissertation, University of California, Los Angeles, 1976.

Part III
HMO of Pennsylvania

12

Introduction

HMO of Pennsylvania is an independent practice association HMO that operates in seven counties in the Philadelphia and Allentown areas.[1] It is a wholly owned for-profit subsidiary of U. S. Healthcare, which was created in 1981, after HMO-PA had become well established, to develop and operate HMOs elsewhere in the country. As we will discuss further in chapter 14, U. S. Healthcare performs important management functions for HMO-PA, and most of its senior managers were transferred from the HMO when the parent company was formed. U. S. Healthcare's second plan, HMO-New Jersey, became operational in March 1983. Its other plans are located in Florida, the Chicago area, and New York City, and it will shortly be operational in Pittsburgh, Delaware, and Connecticut.

By all accounts, HMO of Pennsylvania is one of the real stars of the HMO industry in terms of its performance in the marketplace. Its enrollment in March 1985 totaled some 330,000, making it the largest IPA nationally. In June 1984, the plan had 254,000 enrollees, making it the eighth largest HMO in the country, after three of the Kaiser plans (Northern California, Southern California, and Oregon), Health Insurance Plan (HIP) of Greater New York, Group Health Cooperative of Puget Sound, CIGNA Healthplan of California, and Health Net in California.[2] Furthermore, its growth continues at an accelerated pace, having added 69,000 new members in 1983 and another 93,000 in 1984 (table 12.1).

The plan has also performed well financially. In 1981, HMO-PA generated $469,000 in pretax profits, based on total revenues

Table 12.1

HMO-PA Enrollment Growth,
1979–1985

Year*	Members	Employer Groups
1979	39,000	900
1980	59,000	1,100
1981	87,000	1,500
1982	126,000	1,700
1983	195,000	2,200
1984	288,000	2,900
1985	374,000	3,400

* As of December.

of $31.0 million. By 1984, pretax profits for U. S. Healthcare were $21.3 million on a revenue base of $205.6 million; 70.4 percent of the pretax profits and 77.9 percent of the revenue base are attributed to the Pennsylvania plan.

This report is an account of some of the reasons for the success of HMO-PA. The next chapter characterizes the medical marketplace in which the plan operates. Then, an overview of the plan is presented, dealing with such topics as the role of primary care physicians, hospital and other provider relationships, marketing, utilization control, member services, financial management, and organizational culture. Finally, the key factors that appear to account for the plan's success are discussed.

Notes

1. The seven counties are Bucks, Chester, Delaware, Lehigh, Montgomery, Northampton, and Philadelphia.
2. *Census Preview* (Excelsior, Minn.: InterStudy, 1985).

13

The Market

For years Philadelphia has been regarded as a poor environment for HMOs. It has a stable population with little turnover or net growth; solo, fee-for-service medical practice predominates; patients have formed long-term attachments to physicians; and high Blue Cross discounts for hospital services have given Blue Cross an important edge over competing plans. Yet, when asked about the prevailing wisdom that Philadelphia was not fertile ground for HMO growth, U. S. Healthcare's president, Leonard Abramson, replied, "That's not the prevailing wisdom, that's the prevailing excuse." In this chapter we discuss characteristics of the Philadelphia area that are generally believed to contribute to HMO growth, specifically, demographic factors, medical cost and supply data, and information on competing insurers.

A note on the presentation of data by geographic area is in order. Depending on the statistic in question, data may be available by city, county, state, or metropolitan statistical area (MSA). We have reported data for HMO-PA's seven-county service area where possible; when county data are not available, MSA data are often substituted. The Philadelphia MSA and HMO-PA's service area overlap, but they are not coterminous. The Philadelphia MSA includes Philadelphia, Chester, Bucks, Delaware, and Montgomery counties in Pennsylvania and Burlington, Camden, and Gloucester counties in New Jersey. The service area of HMO-PA includes the five Pennsylvania counties listed above as well as Northampton and Lehigh counties, but not the three New Jersey counties. Other data, unfortunately, are only available for the city of Philadelphia or for the state of Pennsylvania as a whole.

Demographic Characteristics

With respect to the potential for HMO growth, the demographic
characteristics of the Philadelphia area are mixed. It is the fourth
largest metropolitan area in the United States, although its population declined by about 2 percent between 1970 and 1980. The
population of HMO-PA's service area also declined between 1970
and 1980, by almost 4 percent. Philadelphia and Delaware counties accounted for all of this decline (13 and 8 percent, respectively), while the other five counties in the service area grew
(table 13.1).

The seven counties in HMO-PA's service area vary significantly in terms of population size and density. Philadelphia
County is under 140 square miles and averages more than 12,000
people per square mile. By contrast, Chester County is about 760
square miles, with just over 400 people per square mile. Thus, the
service area contains densely populated urban communities (primarily Philadelphia and Delaware counties) plus mostly suburban
areas of varying density.

There are also variations in income, unemployment, and
level of education. Montgomery County, the heart of HMO-PA's
service area and site of U. S. Healthcare's corporate headquarters,
is part of Philadelphia's Main Line. It is an affluent suburban area
with the highest median income ($25,800) and lowest unemploy-
ment (5.2 percent) of the seven counties. Three-quarters of the
county residents are high school graduates. By contrast, Philadelphia County has a median income of $16,400 and an unemploy-
ment rate of 6.9 percent. Just over half of the residents of Philadelphia County are high school graduates. The median family
income in HMO-PA's service area, except for Philadelphia
County, was above the U.S. average of $20,000 in 1980. Except for
Lehigh and Northampton counties, which have suffered from lay-
offs in the steel industry, the unemployment rate for the service
area is lower than the U.S. average of 7.2 percent (November
1984).

The data presented so far support the notion that the Philadelphia area is fertile for HMO development. However, Pennsylvania is a highly unionized state, and access to union workers
depends on union as well as employer interest in an HMO alternative. Thirty-three percent of the Pennsylvania work force is unionized, compared to 23 percent for the United States as a whole
(1980). Data on union membership in the Philadelphia area are
not readily available.

Table 13.1

Selected Demographic Characteristics of the HMO-PA Service Area

County	1980 Population	Change Since 1970 (%)	Median Family Income, 1979 ($)	Unemployment Rate November, 1984 (%)	High School Graduates, 1980 (%)
Philadelphia	1,688,210	−13.4	16,388	6.9	54.2
Montgomery	643,621	3.1	25,803	5.2	75.8
Delaware	557,007	− 8.0	23,103	5.3	72.3
Bucks	479,211	15.0	24,402	7.1	74.7
Chester	316,660	14.0	25,533	5.3	76.4
Lehigh	272,349	6.7	21,906	7.4	64.5
Northampton	225,418	5.1	21,333	9.3	61.7
Total	4,180,476				
U.S. Average		− 3.7	19,917	7.2	66.5

Sources: U.S. Department of Commerce, Bureau of the Census, Statistical Abstract of the United States, 1984 (Washington, D.C.: Government Printing Office, 1983) and County and City Data Book—1983 (Washington, D.C.: Government Printing Office, 1983); U.S. Department of Labor, Bureau of Labor Statistics, personal communication.

Finally, the age distribution in the Philadelphia MSA is slightly older than the norm for all MSAs, which explains part of the higher-than-average hospital cost and utilization highlighted in the next section.

Medical Cost and Supply Factors

Medical cost and supply data for the Philadelphia area indicate a favorable environment for HMO growth. Philadelphia is a high-cost, high-utilizing area with an oversupply of hospital beds and physicians. In this environment, an efficient delivery system offering more benefits at a lower cost is likely to attract employer and employee interest.

One important indicator is the cost of hospital care. Average annual inpatient expenses per capita for the Philadelphia MSA were $431 in 1980, 12 percent higher than the average of $386 for all MSAs. One reason for this is higher utilization of hospital care; there were 1,380 inpatient days per thousand persons in the Philadelphia MSA in 1981, compared to 1,270 days per thousand for all MSAs. Admission rates are about average, but the average length of stay in 1983 was 9.0 days, compared to the national figure of 7.6 days.

The supply of hospital beds in Philadelphia is approximately equal to MSA norms. In 1981, there were 4.53 beds per thousand persons in the Philadelphia MSA, compared to a national MSA average of 4.48. However, the occupancy rate in Philadelphia (81 percent) is higher than the average of all MSAs (76 percent), reflecting higher utilization.

The area also has high physician-population ratios. The number of nonfederal medical doctors (M.D.'s) per thousand persons in HMO-PA's service area was 2.9 in 1981, compared to a national average of 2.1 (table 13.2). This ratio varies by county, from 1.3 M.D.'s per thousand in Bucks to 4.0 in Montgomery. Although county-specific data on D.O.'s are not available, there were 2,860 D.O.'s in Pennsylvania in 1984; Philadelphia is known to have a high concentration of D.O.'s because the Philadelphia College of Osteopathic Medicine is located there. This concentration is reflected in the fact that approximately 40 percent of HMO-PA's participating primary care physicians are D.O.'s.

While these data imply that HMOs might have relatively easy access to physician services, there are two factors that could have a countervailing effect. First, there are six medical schools

Table 13.2

Physician-Population Ratios in the
HMO-PA Service Area

County	1981 Population*	Nonfederal† M.D.'s, 1981	M.D.'s per 1,000 Persons
Philadelphia	1,672,459	6,236	3.7
Montgomery	649,177	2,565	4.0
Delaware	551,582	1,217	2.2
Bucks	488,787	620	1.3
Chester	322,151	472	1.5
Lehigh	274,285	550	2.0
Northampton	227,073	394	1.7
Total	4,185,514	12,054	2.9

* *Source:* Federal-State Cooperative Program for Population Estimates (U.S. Bureau of the Census and Pennsylvania State Data Center, Middletown).

† *Source:* American Medical Association.

in the area, so many teaching physicians are not in full-time private practice. Second, few physicians in the MSA practice in groups: in 1980, 16 percent of them did, compared to the 23 percent national MSA average. The prevalence of solo or small partnership practice is not necessarily a hindrance to the establishment of IPA-model HMOs, although it is clearly a barrier to the formation of other models.

Health Insurance

A final key element of the market is the nature of competing indemnity carriers and prepaid health plans. Around Philadelphia, Blue Cross accounts for about 70 percent of the privately insured market. Blue Cross pays hospitals on the basis of their costs, which average more than 20 percent below full billed charges. This deep discount helps explain Blue Cross' sizable share of the market and the small share of commercial health insurers, who must reflect in their premiums the fact that they pay full charges.

There are three other HMOs in the Philadelphia area, each with approximately 30,000 members as of June 1984 (table 13.3). The Health Service Plan of Pennsylvania is a group model, Philadelphia Health Plan is a network, and Delaware Valley HMO is an IPA. All have been operational for several years, yet only HMO-PA has shown significant growth in enrollment. Competition may intensify in the near future, however, because each of the other

Table 13.3

HMOs in the Philadelphia Area

Plan	Year Formed	Model	Members June 1980	Members June 1984
HMO of Pennsylvania Blue Bell	1976	IPA	47,664	254,195
Health America-Health Service Plan of Pennsylvania Philadelphia	1974	Group	19,600	31,618
Philadelphia Health Plan Philadelphia	1974	Network	23,715	30,016
Delaware Valley HMO Concordville	1978	IPA	6,430	27,497

Sources: Modified from InterStudy, *Census Preview* (Excelsior, Minn.: InterStudy, 1985) and *HMO Growth, 1980–81* (Excelsior, Minn.: InterStudy, 1982).

three plans has changed, or is considering a change, to for-profit status.

Summary

On balance, factors favorable to HMO development in the Philadelphia area override the few negative characteristics. Although the metropolitan area is not growing overall, it is still the fourth largest in the United States. Furthermore, residents of the suburban counties that comprise the mainstay of HMO-PA's service area are affluent and well educated, and their numbers are growing. Most important, there are enough M.D.'s and D.O.'s to allow HMOs to recruit physicians, and hospital costs and utilization are high, permitting HMOs to achieve savings. Furthermore, despite significant Blue Cross penetration of the market, the competitive situation is not particularly threatening. Relatively little commercial insurance is sold for hospital coverage, and the three other HMOs in the area have not penetrated the market to any great extent. Only HMO-PA has capitalized on the opportunities for HMO growth offered by the market conditions in Philadelphia.

14

Overview

The predecessor of HMO-PA, Family Medical Care, Inc. (FMC), began operations in 1974. FMC was a nonprofit IPA owned by R.H. Medical Services, Inc., a proprietary hospital company. Between 1975 and 1977, FMC and its successor, HMO-PA, received feasibility and planning and development grants totaling about $815,000 from what was then the U.S. Department of Health, Education and Welfare.

In 1977, HMO-PA was formed in order to purchase FMC: HMO-PA thus acquired FMC's assets and about 1,200 members for just over $500,000. Leonard Abramson, executive director of FMC and vice president of R.H. Medical Services, became president of HMO-PA; he continues as president of U.S. Healthcare. At about the same time, the plan became federally qualified and received a federal loan of $2.5 million to fund projected operating deficits over the subsequent five years.

After 1977, enrollment grew quickly, and by 1980 HMO-PA was well in the black. In 1981, the company decided to reorganize as a for-profit entity. In mid-1981, United States Health Care Systems, Inc. (USHCSI) was formed. The venture capital firm of E.M. Warburg, Pincus, and Co., Inc., of New York provided much of the capital, and USHCSI made arrangements for settling the outstanding HMO-PA debt with the federal government.

Thus U. S. Healthcare, as USHCSI was renamed in 1985, acquired the assets, liabilities, and operations of HMO-PA; it also acquired the HMO-PA name for business purposes. HMO-PA is the oldest and largest of the plans owned and operated by U. S. Healthcare.[1]

With the challenge of running several HMOs, U. S. Healthcare management has faced decisions about which functions to
centralize and which to decentralize. In general, the preference is
for centralization, in order to improve efficiency and to create a
corporationwide perspective. Many systems are standardized, and
most U. S. Healthcare departments have full-time training staff
who travel to new locations and orient employees. Employees,
too, are encouraged to have a corporate perspective. New sales
force recruits, for example, are told during the hiring process that
they may be transferred to any of U. S. Healthcare's locations.

Functions centralized at corporate headquarters in Blue Bell,
Pennsylvania, include

— Claims processing

— Enrollment

— Finance

— Personnel (most functions)

Functions that are by and large decentralized—although employees are trained by U. S. Healthcare or HMO-PA personnel, or
both—include marketing, member services, and provider relations.

The distribution of responsibilities and staff between the
corporate parent and its subsidiaries is still evolving. The overlap
between U. S. Healthcare and HMO-PA is the greatest, for historical reasons. As new and geographically more distant plans become operational, a more regional system may evolve. It is clear,
however, that the organizational structure as it now exists has
been carefully conceived and that, as will become obvious in
later chapters, very little that happens in this organization occurs
by accident.

HMO-PA offers a single, comprehensive benefit package that
covers all preventive care, outpatient visits, inpatient care, maternity services, emergencies, and limited mental health, substance
abuse, and home care services. Hospitalization is unlimited except for psychiatric care (35 days) and drug and alcohol treatment
(acute phase only). There is a $2.00 copayment for outpatient vis-
its to primary care physicians; copayments are higher for emergency visits, mental health counseling after two free visits, and
physician visits to the home. There is no cost sharing for referred
specialty care. At the employer's option, a rider for the prescription drug benefit can be purchased to supplement the basic plan;

copayments are $2.50 per prescription or refill. Home care is covered only as an alternative to hospital care. Dental services are not provided, other than preventive care for children under age 12. HMO-PA uses straight community rating to establish its premiums, that is, it does not use the flexibility in federal law that allows federally qualified HMOs to adjust premiums based on a group's age, sex, occupational code, or other objectively measured characteristics. The plan does not have any Medicaid enrollees. It has only a few thousand Medicare members, for whom it is reimbursed on a cost basis, but it intends to seek a Medicare risk contract. It plans to limit Medicare enrollment to 5 percent of the total.

Relations With Providers

Primary Care Physicians

Primary care physicians are the key to HMO-PA's delivery system. They deliver all primary care, refer for specialty and hospital services (and thereby determine the resulting expense for these services), and have ongoing contact with current and prospective HMO members. As a result, HMO-PA pays considerable attention to the selection of these physicians. Good relations with primary care physicians are also important because satisfied physicians will both keep current enrollees happy and attract new members to the plan. Relations between primary care physicians and the HMO have generally been excellent. Stringent selection criteria, physician risk sharing, attractive remuneration levels, and good communication between HMO-PA and its IPA have worked to control utilization and build good relations. This has not occurred by chance, but rather because HMO-PA management has made relations with primary care physicians one of its highest priorities.

Under contract with HMO-PA are about 560 primary care physicians practicing in 359 different offices. The physicians have their own association, which constitutes the IPA. Primary care physicians at HMO-PA can be internists, family practitioners, or pediatricians, and they can be either M.D.'s or D.O.'s. Obstetricians and gynecologists are considered specialists and cannot join the IPA. Some 60 percent of primary care physicians are M.D.'s, the majority of them family practitioners; the remaining 40 percent are D.O.'s. Many of the physicians are in solo practice; groups are typically small, rarely exceeding three or four physicians. Each physician must be willing and able to accept at least 500 HMO patients. Panel size varies widely and may reach as many as 2,000 HMO patients per physician, which might represent 60 to 70 percent of a typical practice.

In the remainder of this section, we describe HMO-PA's relationship with its primary care physicians, including the physician selection and recertification processes, risk-sharing arrangements with physicians, and methods of communication and provider education.

Selection and Recertification. Initially, HMO-PA had some difficulty recruiting physicians, but this situation has changed dramatically over the last eight years. Certain parts of the service area have always been more resistant than others, but there are now very few towns in which recruitment is a problem.

The selection process and required annual recertification of primary care physicians are important features of HMO-PA. Selection criteria, which have been revised over time, are adhered to strictly and cover the following:

— State licensure

— Malpractice insurance

— Office standards (for example, at least two examination rooms, adequate waiting area, and an electrocardiograph in nonpediatric offices)

— Adequate office hours and 24-hour coverage, with a response time of no more than 30 minutes in emergencies

— Privileges at a participating hospital

— Proficiency in various specified procedures (such as minor surgery, visual screening, tonometry, and sigmoidoscopy)

— Ability to accept at least 500 HMO patients and a scheduling policy for all patients of no more than five patients per hour.

— In good standing professionally and either board certified or eligible for certification

Prospective primary care physicians first complete an application and supply much of the above information in writing. Next, a member of the provider relations staff visits the office to observe its location and physical appearance, review the appointment book, and interview the physician to explain HMO-PA in more detail. After certain data provided on the application form are verified, applicants who appear to meet the criteria are interviewed by one of HMO-PA's medical directors. An important purpose of the interview is to determine whether applicants are supportive of the philosophy and concept of an IPA-type HMO. Applicants are also requested to bring several medical charts, which serve as a basis for discussing patterns of practice with the medical director. References may be required.

There is typically a backlog of physician applications, and 20 to 40 percent of initial applications are denied. Common reasons for denial include lack of privileges at a participating hospital and failure to meet the plan's standards of office practice regarding scheduling and comprehensiveness of services.

If the criteria for membership are met, a physician may be admitted provisionally to the IPA. After a two-year probationary period, he or she becomes a full-fledged IPA member. After the probationary period, all offices are recertified on an annual basis. It should be noted that there is no provision in the contract between HMO-PA and the primary care physicians requiring exclusivity; physicians may participate in, for example, the nearby Delaware Valley IPA as well, although few have done so. In addition, not all physicians in a group practice must join HMO-PA, although participation by all members of the group is preferred.

The annual recertification process includes the following:

— A site visit by a member of the provider relations staff to check for neat, professional atmosphere and compliance with criteria for office standards

— Review of practice statistics with the physician comparing his or her practice with the IPA average (for example, number of referrals per visit, amount left in specialty fund, use of participating versus nonparticipating specialists, total hospital charges, use of participating versus nonparticipating hospitals)

— Review by a medical director of grievances filed against the office (the norm for nonprocedural complaints is two or fewer per year)

— A written survey of at least one-third of an office's subscribers to assess their satisfaction in terms of waiting time for appointments, waiting time in the office, and overall impression of the care and service received

— A surprise check on physician availability and response
time to off-hours calls (HMO-PA staff call on a weekend
or at night, and the physician has a maximum of two
chances to respond within 30 minutes)

Approximately 5 to 10 percent of recertifications are denied initially, but almost all of the physicians in question correct the
problem and retain their membership. The typical sanction for
noncomplying physicians is a freeze on new patients, meaning
that no new HMO members will be sent to him or her.

Risk Sharing. The reimbursement formulas reflect the economic model of the plan, which is viewed as critical to its performance. Central to that model is the reimbursement of the primary
care physicians, who are capitated for their own services and are
either individually or collectively at risk for most referred services. The potential bonus to physicians for efficient utilization can
be a significant amount; however, it is subject to the annual recertification procedure by the medical directors, which includes
passing a quality assurance review. The potential loss for excess
utilization is restricted to 20 percent of the monthly capitation.

Three pools are established to pay for physician and hospital
services, The first pool is for primary care physicians. A capitation amount that varies with patient age (0–1, 2–11, 12–20, 21 and
over, and Medicare beneficiaries) is established. The full capitation amount averaged $8.13 per month for non-Medicare mem-
bers in 1985, ranging from $5.80 (for a patient age 12–20) to $19.84
(for the first 24 months of life). Each month the primary physician
receives 80 percent of the capitation amount and is also allowed
to collect a copayment of $2 per visit. The remaining 20 percent is
withheld to cover deficits in the specialist pool, as described below.

The second pool is for specialized care. Each primary care
physician is assigned a target dollar amount, which varies with
patient age, for specialist care. Expenses for specialist and other
referral services (such as laboratory services) are charged against
the primary care physician's individual account; however, a cata-
strophic risk pool provides partial protection for very expensive
cases. Any primary care physician with a surplus in his or her
specialist account at the end of the six-month reconciliation period keeps the surplus. In contrast, deficits are not charged
against the individual physician; rather, they are shared among
all primary physicians (including those with a surplus) and are
paid from the 20 percent withheld. In a typical year, about half of

the physicians have a surplus, and the accumulated deficits from the remaining half consume about half of the 20 percent withheld.

Finally, a hospital pool is established and targets assigned to individual primary care physicians. Those who have a surplus share it fifty-fifty with the HMO. The HMO absorbs all losses, but few physicians run a loss. Some physicians receive bonuses of several thousand dollars each year for unused hospital funds.

The minimum a primary care physician can receive under this system is around $25 a visit. This assumes that he or she receives only 80 percent of the capitation amount, plus the $2 per visit copayment. Using HMO-PA's 1985 composite assumption of 3.4 encounters per patient per year, the minimum 80 percent capitation (excluding bonuses) for a physician with 1,000 patients would be about $78,000. A physician who receives the full capitation along with the bonuses distributed based on panel size can receive some 20 to 40 percent over the minimum, which is signficantly above what he or she would expect in the fee-for-service system.

The medical directors review the surpluses generated by individual physicians or groups of physicians, and a pattern of consistently high surpluses would alert them to the possibility of underservice. Physicians with high surpluses are carefully scrutinized; however, the medical directors report that high surpluses are not correlated with lower quality of care.

Relations with Physicians. Management goes to great lengths to maintain good relations with primary care physicians by understanding and meeting their needs to the greatest extent possible. Both physician leadership and HMO efforts to support and communicate with physicians are important components of HMO-PA's business strategy.

There are two full-time senior medical directors, both of whom are former primary care physicians, and four part-time associate medical directors. All six continue to have private practices. A committee structure has been created to facilitate physician input into management decision making. There are four major committees: executive, membership, peer review, and quality assurance.

— *The executive committee* is composed of 12 physicians elected by the IPA membership, plus the senior medical directors as ex-officio members. This committee oversees medical delivery and advises HMO-PA management on provider relations issues. It also appoints IPA physicians to the membership and peer review committees, delegates tasks to these committees, and reviews their findings.

— *The membership committee* reviews all physicians' applications.

— *The peer review committee* handles problems or complaints about individual physicians and recommends further action to the executive committee.

— *The quality assurance committee,* composed of the five medical directors and selected HMO staff members, meets monthly to approve office recertifications and deal with other medical delivery issues, such as coverage policy.

Every effort is made by HMO-PA to educate physicians about HMO policies and procedures, to respond to their questions and concerns, and to provide services to facilitate their practice of medicine. This reflects the philosophy that a satisfied physician will translate into satisfied HMO patients. HMO-PA's provider relations staff numbers 18, in addition to the 6 medical directors. The following are examples of HMO-PA provider relations initiatives:

— *Physician office coordinator program:* HMO-PA holds training sessions for physicians' office managers or administrative assistants to help them with practice management techniques and HMO procedures. Some office supplies and marketing materials are provided—for example, stickers with red apples (the HMO's symbol) to identify the medical records of HMO patients and brochures on special HMO-PA programs.

— *Provider relations territories:* HMO-PA provider relations staff have territories which they service, primarily by handling telephone requests for information or assistance.

— *Medical director visits:* One of the medical directors visits each office at least annually, more often for large practices.

— *Primary care physician newsletter:* A monthly publication is distributed to update physicians on new programs, staff changes, results of committee meetings, and so on.

— *Recruitment of new associates:* HMO-PA will advertise in medical journals and "play matchmaker" to help physicians recruit associates. The plan will also provide loans and other support for recent medical school graduates who are willing to establish independent practices in parts of HMO-PA's service area where the plan has had difficulty recruiting.

Specialists

More than 3,800 specialists have contractual agreements with HMO-PA. Since primary care physicians act as gatekeepers, HMO-PA does not seek to limit the pool of participating specialists; rather, it tries to recruit specialists used by its primary care physicians in order to preserve existing referral patterns.

Participating specialists must agree to HMO-PA's maximum reimbursement levels and meet certain criteria. The criteria are not as extensive as those for primary care physicians, but they address many of the same areas (board certification or eligibility, malpractice insurance, adequate office hours, and so on). The maximum reimbursement amount, called REF (respectable, equitable fees) by the HMO, is intended to approximate Medicare payment levels. The REF is reviewed at least annually.

The HMO generally tries to pay nonparticipating specialists no more than the REF for participating specialists. However, because the plan guarantees that enrollees will not be financially liable for more than the copayments, the full billed rate is paid if the specialist insists. No specialist is reimbursed by the plan without a written referral from the primary care physician. Since these billings are charged against the primary care physician's individual account, as described above, one incentive to refer only to participating specialists is the knowledge that scheduled payment levels will not be exceeded. Of HMO-PA's total payments for specialty care in 1984, about 90 percent went to participating specialists.

Participating specialists are encouraged to use what HMO-PA terms its "cost-effective programs." These programs are a mechanism for sharing the savings from reduced utilization with physicians. The largest and most visible is the L'il Appleseed program to promote early obstetrical discharges. If a member's obstetrician and pediatrician determine there is no risk, and if the patient herself wants to, she can be discharged two days after a normal delivery and four days after a Cesarean section. With early discharge, the mother receives a home visit from a pediatric nurse, a package of educational materials, and a $75 check to pay for in-home services. The obstetrician receives $75 and the pediatrician $25, both in addition to normal fees. Approximately 80 to 85 percent of all maternity patients participate in the program. Surveys of participants show that mothers are enthusiastic about Li'l Appleseed. Similar programs exist to share the savings from reduced hospital costs with other specialists, such as by substituting home health care for inpatient care (through a hospice program or house calls), performing vasectomies as office procedures, and substituting ambulatory for inpatient surgery.

Hospitals

HMO-PA has contractual arrangements with 62 hospitals, which are generally reimbursed on a negotiated per diem basis. The per diems average roughly 20 percent below full billed charges and approximately 5 to 10 percent above what Blue Cross pays. HMO-PA contracts primarily with community hospitals and does not view hospital choice as a marketing tool, believing instead that potential enrollees are attracted by physicians and are comfortable letting their physician choose the hospital. Hospitals thus are selected by HMO-PA largely on the basis of their willingness to accept negotiated rates that will allow the plan to price its benefits competitively. For example, HMO-PA does not contract with certain prestigious teaching hospitals unless these hospitals reduce their prices to acceptable levels.

For 11 procedures that account for between 40 and 50 percent of admissions, the HMO has developed and implemented in several hospitals its own prospective payment system. Under that system, a target length of stay by diagnosis is established, as well as high and low cut-off, or trim, points. The trim points are conceptually similar to those used to determine "outliers" in the Medicare prospective payment system, except that they apply to the average of all patients for a diagnosis at each hospital rather than to each patient. Between the trim points, the hospital receives a payment that equals the negotiated per diem at that hospital multiplied by the target length of stay. Retrospective adjustments are made for stays of average duration at a particular hospital that fall outside the ranges established by the trim points. Currently, targets and payments vary by hospital, but the plan is seeking to move to a single norm. Savings to date have been significant. For example, the cost of open-heart surgery has been reduced from between $25,000 and $27,000 to between $15,000 and $16,000 per case for hospital and physician fees combined

Hospital utilization is controlled in a number of ways. While there is no formal precertification process, the primary care physicians are given incentives to be conservative in their use of the hospital, and any admission by a specialist requires approval of the referring primary care physician. In addition, hospitals are required to notify the plan of all admissions. Similarly, in lieu of the typical concurrent review, lists of hospitalized patients, along with their diagnoses and dates of admission, are posted on a board and monitored daily; statistics are assembled at the end of each month and used to track overall hospital utilization. A small home care department with two registered nurses reviews both questionable admissions and extended stays, working with physicians to explore alternative treatments.

Other Providers

HMO-PA has developed imaginative relationships with a number of other providers. Doing so exemplifies the plan's willingness to innovate and use its economic clout by engaging in volume purchasing from a limited number of providers who are forced to compete for contracts. First, the plan has agreements with a large number of *pharmacies*. All outpatient prescription drug costs are fully capitated by the pharmacy, and each plan enrollee with drug coverage selects a participating pharmacy for prescriptions. In addition, the plan has partially implemented capitation for *radiology* and *podiatry* services; ultimately these services will be capitated for all primary care physicians' offices. *Laboratory* and *mental health* services are also capitated. For mental health services each primary physician (not the patient) selects a psychiatrist, or group of psychiatrists, who are at risk for both inpatient and outpatient mental health services. Because mental health services are prepaid, the primary care physicians have an incentive to refer patients and psychiatrists have an incentive to be conservative in their use of the hospital.

The history of the capitation for mental health services is instructive. Before capitation, the plan was experiencing 50 to 55 psychiatric inpatient days per thousand members. A closer look revealed that the average length of stay was nearly 30 days (with a benefit limit of 35 days) and that hospitalizations occurred disproportionately near the end of a benefit year, after 18 or 19 outpatient visits had been used (with a benefit limit of 20 visits). As a result, HMO-PA changed the basis of payment from fee-for-service to a negotiated capitation and reduced the number of mental health providers from over 400 individuals to just 15 groups. Nearly two years later, the average length of stay is nine days, and total inpatient days per thousand are about 22. The medical directors believe the quality of care has improved as well, now that providers work harder on an outpatient basis to keep patients well.

Another example of HMO-PA's changing relationships with providers is its method of paying *ambulatory surgery centers*. In the past, the plan has not pushed ambulatory surgery and has found facility fees to vary between $400 and $1,200 a procedure. By negotiating rates and placing a limit on payment, it believes that annual savings in excess of $500,000 can be attained.

Finally, the plan has entered into *full-risk capitation contracts* with two prominent teaching hospitals (or, more precisely, with the separate legal entities each of the hospitals has established) for services to approximately 12,000 HMO-PA members. These contracts evolved in part because of frustration with the hospitals' faculty practice plans, which did not have efficient utilization patterns and thus operated at a loss, which was largely borne by other primary care physicians and the HMO.

Under full-risk capitation, the capitated organization receives 82 percent of premiums on behalf of enrollees. This approximates the percentage of the premium dollar in the plan as a whole that is allocated to medical care (with the balance being allocated to administration, marketing, and profits). The organization develops its own system of controls and rewards for physicians. One of the problems with the primary care physicians associated with those organizations in the past has been that they tended to lose track of patients once the patients had been referred to specialists; the hospitals now have an incentive to work with the doctors to reduce the likelihood that that will happen. HMO-PA says hospital utilization in these practices dropped 30 percent after the new arrangement was instituted.

Similar agreements have recently been negotiated with two other hospitals in Philadelphia and with four physicians' offices in Allentown.

Utilization Control Mechanisms

Utilization of all medical services, but especially of hospital and specialty care, is controlled in a variety of ways. HMO-PA uses a combination of financial incentives, administrative requirements, and physician education and feedback to achieve its utilization targets. Management has deliberately avoided trying to standardize the practice of medicine; this bias against "cookbook medicine" stems from the view that physicians know how to practice before they join the IPA. As most of HMO-PA's incentive programs have already been described, this section focuses on administrative controls and physician feedback.

Administrative procedures for utilization review include the following requirements:

— Written referral from the primary care physician for specialty care

— HMO-PA notification of all admissions

— No Friday or Saturday admissions for elective surgery

— Ambulatory surgery for certain procedures

Methods of educating physicians so they can better control utilization include

— Visits to primary care physicians' offices by provider relations staff at least once a year to discuss practice patterns

— Monthly management reports to primary care physicians with data on

number of members in the practice

total capitation funds received

amount of money in the 20 percent withholding pool

number of office visits and comparison with the HMO average

average amount of money received per visit

number of specialty referrals and comparison with the HMO average (as a percentage of all visits)

hospital admissions and days of care, and comparison of inpatient use rates with the HMO average

— Dissemination of information on the plan's early discharge programs

— Assistance from home care department for physicians seeking alternatives to hospital care

It is worth noting that HMO-PA has elected *not* to institute certain measures. For example, it makes no systematic attempt to identify and distribute recent literature on patient outcome studies that supports early hospital discharge. In addition, there are no treatment protocols for common problems, no standards for diagnostic testing or screening, no closed drug formulary, and so forth. There are two reasons for the lack of clinical standards. First, HMO-PA wishes to avoid a "min-max" relationship with physicians: if the HMO decreed minimum quality standards, then those could be exactly what inpatients received. Second, HMO-PA prefers to rely on financial incentives rather than administrative controls whenever possible. Also, since radiology, mental health, pharmacy, and other services are capitated, there is less need for HMO-PA to impose controls on utilization of those services.

Marketing

Leonard Abramson views marketing as one of the most important factors in the HMO's success. HMO-PA was repeatedly described as "market driven." Its marketing strategy is carefully conceived and highly systematized, with little left to chance. Systematization is reflected in

— A high degree of computerization and reliance on quantitative measures of staff performance

— Extensive staff training programs

— Careful attention to the integration of steps needed to market, first to employers and then to employees, followed by measures to assure that new members understand and are comfortable with the plan and the delivery system

— A commitment to having satisfied enrollees, reflecting the view that word of mouth is the most effective form of advertising

The linchpin of the marketing strategy is a carefully selected, trained, and organized sales force. The plan also spends $2 million annually (roughly 1 percent of revenues) on advertising, including television, newspaper, and billboard ads. The same symbols—an apple and the color red—are used consistently in promotional efforts. (For example, the sales representatives wear red blazers as do actors in the television commercials.)

Marketing starts with the identification of new employer groups to approach. An individual on the telemarketing staff calls prospective groups to elicit information on the nature of the business, the health plans currently offered, premium rates and how premium costs are shared between the firm and employees, and the renewal date of the indemnity plan contract. If feasible, candidate groups are assessed to determine if there is any reason not to approach them, perhaps because the group is likely to have high medical costs, (for example, an asbestos factory) or because the employer contribution to premiums is so low that few employees would be willing to pay the difference for HMO coverage.

A sales representative then approaches the groups, typically several months in advance of the contract renewal date or open season for the employer's indemnity plan. These sales representatives are carefully selected and undergo extensive training. Of 100 resumes reviewed, 10 persons, on average, are invited for interviews, and only one is offered a position. The interviewing process is elaborate and usually requires the candidate to spend a day making calls with a sales representative, mostly to ensure that the candidate is fully informed about the nature of the job before accepting it.

During the five-week training program, a class of 10 to 15 prospective representatives will attend classroom sessions, meet with each HMO department head, role-play (both one-on-one presentations to benefit managers and group presentations to employees), and travel with sales representatives. An important reason for the training process is to ensure that sales representatives know the product well and can clearly articulate the benefits and how one goes about getting them. Self-study guides have been prepared, and there are frequent review sessions and quizzes. After training, each sales representative is assigned a territory and a quota; remuneration depends in large part on achieving and surpassing the quota.

A series of well-defined steps is generally followed in marketing to employers. These include formal presentations and extensive written materials that are distributed at the workplace and mailed to the home. In addition, the sales representative tries to meet with new enrollees. At those meetings, emphasis is placed on such topics as the role of the primary care physician as case manager, what to do in case of an emergency, and how to use the member relations department for questions or problems. In addition, the member relations department phones each new member and makes sure that a primary care physician and a pharmacy have been selected. The plan believes that member satisfaction is a major contributor to plan growth; staying in touch with the customer is engrained in the organization's philosophy.

Member Services

The member services department has been important to HMO-PA from its inception, and it is highly visible within the organization. Its major functions are to solve individual problems and to highlight problem areas throughout the organization, creating a feedback loop. In order to facilitate problem solving for members, efforts are made to answer all questions over the telephone—letter writing is encouraged only as a last resort. The department supplies members with form letters for filing formal grievances.

The member services staff, which handles calls for both the Pennsylvania and the New Jersey plans, consists of a director and 27 full-time-equivalent member service supervisors and representatives. As of December 1984, the average number of calls received by the department was 1,600 per day; an experienced representative is expected to handle at least 70 per day. Supervisors monitor the service representatives every six months by listening to random calls in order to evaluate the representatives for response time, courtesy, and understanding of the caller's problem.

Member services staff seek to respond in a personal, accurate, yet low-cost way. The department relies on a combination of technology and specialization to handle the rapidly increasing number of inquiries efficiently. On the technological side, a sophisticated computerized telephone system automatically sends each call to the first available representative and records the average waiting time. If no representative is free to take a call, a taped message will respond. At peak times, the average wait is about two to three minutes; the goal is never to use the taped message. Still under development is a plan to give each representative a computer terminal with access to the 100 most common questions that members ask. When the representative answers the phone, he or she will be able to call up the question and the correct answer on the screen. The ability to read answers off the screen will, it is hoped, both increase accuracy and reduce response time.

When the computer system becomes operational, representatives will be divided between those who take common questions and read answers off the screeen and those who handle questions requiring research. The common-problems representatives will be instructed to take the names and numbers of callers with more unusual questions; research representatives will produce answers for these calls within 24 hours. Research representatives may be further specialized into claims researchers, enrollment researchers, and so forth. Another form of specialization occurred when provider calls were transferred to the provider relations department; member services no longer handles calls from specialists, hospitals, or other providers.

Member services also interacts with other departments, both by advising them of policies or procedures that are confusing to members or are causing other problems and by encouraging the other departments to notify member services promptly of any glitches that are likely to provoke calls. Member services tabulates calls received by type of problem and makes these data available to the rest of the organization. The volume of calls by problem area varies from month to month, but the two biggest trouble spots are, typically, enrollment and claims.

Management and Administrative Cost Controls

Adminstrative costs receive considerable attention, and budgets are examined monthly. Also, heavy emphasis is placed on work planning, and managers are required to prepare monthly, annual, and five-year plans, which are reviewed regularly. In addition, the financial staff has developed computer-based financial models to estimate the impact of alternative scenarios (for example, changes in enrollment or costs) and to undertake contingency planning.

Another characteristic of the HMO is its reliance on computers, which are operated around the clock. Equipment has been updated on several occasions, and system changes are constantly being made. The entire staff has a computer orientation, and the system staff has a strong user orientation. Use of the computer starts with the development of the prospects file by the telemarketing staff. Once an employer agrees to offer the plan, a group and membership (enrollment) file is created; this is used for billings, handling of enrollee inquiries, statistical analyses, and so forth. Also on computer files are primary care physicians, specialists, and hospitals (for payment and medical evaluation), claims and encounter data, and various administrative files (such as personnel and accounting).

Claims incurred but not reported, a major financial control problem for some HMOs, are carefully tracked. Hospital expenses are estimated at the time of the hospitalization itself. Specialty claims are estimated statistically on the basis of past patterns that reflect the time lags between date of the service and receipt of claim.

The compensation scheme is designed to tie employees to the objectives of the organization. Senior executives receive stock options, and all employees receive an annual cash bonus if overall corporate goals are met. There is also a separate incentive plan for senior executives if profits exceed those budgeted; the plan is a combination of cash (50 percent) and stock (50 percent). Finally, bonuses are given to employees who make suggestions that are implemented.

Nonfinancial approaches to motivate staff are also important. Open lines of communication are stressed, and senior management is in touch with employees. The personnel department periodically conducts focus groups of three to four employees to discuss problems or just to provide an opportunity for getting better acquainted. A management brainstorming retreat for department heads and senior executives is held once a year, and each attendee is asked to bring at least one new idea.

Organizational Culture and Business Philosophy

A coherent organizational culture and a consistent business philosophy emanate from top management of U. S. Healthcare and HMO-PA. Management is results-oriented and sets quantitative objectives for staff, who display a can-do attitude toward their work. The company's objectives, in order of priority, are

— To provide service to customers

— To maintain good relations with primary care physicians

— To keep employees satisfied and motivated

Both continuity of leadership and the practice of promoting from within have facilitated the diffusion of top management's philosophy throughout the organization. Most of U. S. Healthcare's top managers have been with the firm for several years, and many middle managers have risen from entry-level positions.

The basic tenets of top management at U. S. Healthcare have been effectively communicated to personnel at other levels. The customer service imperative and the importance of good provider relations, in particular, were repeatedly and independently articulated in many different interviews.

This consistency of approach exists at all levels and cuts across all functions. For example, all departments emphasize staff development. Most departments have full-time trainers who started in operations at HMO-PA and now are responsible for training new staff in other U. S. Healthcare locations. There is also a focus on productivity throughout the organization; productivity standards have been developed for claims processors, marketing representatives, and member service representatives. Performance is monitored. Spot checks are made on all aspects of the business that affect customer relations.

Every department has clearly articulated goals for improving its operations, and most of these are quantified. In member services, the goal is to reduce the waiting time for callers to the point where a taped message is never used. In enrollment, the goal is to get enrollment cards to members within two weeks. In marketing, the goal is to enroll 70,000 new subscribers (net) in 1985.

Note

1. The development of HMO-PA is covered in greater detail in two case studies sponsored by the Office of Health Maintenance Organizations: Robert C. Gettys, *Private Sector Investment in Health Maintenance Organizations: A Case Study of Venture Capital Financing*, DHHS publication no. (PHS) 82-50184 (Washington, D.C.: Government Printing Office, 1982), and American Association of Foundations for Medical Care and Office of Health Maintenance Organizations, *HMO of Pennsylvania: A Case Study of an IPA*, DHHS publication no. (PHS) 81-50129 (Washington, D.C.: Government Printing Office, n.d.).

15

Success Factors

During our visit, Abramson articulated five major reasons for HMO-PA's success: location, management (including general administration, marketing, provider relations, and human resources), customer service, innovative programs, and competitive pricing. Of these, we would highlight marketing and relations with primary care physicians as particularly impressive features of HMO-PA. These, in addition to prudent purchasing of medical care, general management, and other, more intangible, factors are discussed below.

Marketing

Marketing is one of HMO-PA's greatest strengths, on two levels. On the micro level, the marketing department is extremely proficient. In terms of strategy, identification of prospects, sales presentation, and account servicing, the plan does an outstanding job, as evidenced by enrollment growth.

On a more global level, marketing is what much of HMO-PA is all about. The company effectively markets itself to the public, to employers, to providers, and to its own employees. A symbol of this approach is the ubiquitous red apple. Many key functions have a strong marketing orientation. This is particularly evident in the well-run provider relations and member service areas; primary physicians and members are seen as customers whose convenience and satisfaction should be maximized. In addition, the Healthy Outlook programs offered to members and employees promote health and serve as potentially powerful marketing tools. Indeed, marketing is far more than selling, it is also having satisfied enrollees who stay with the plan and encourage their neighbors and co-workers to join. An important index of success is the low voluntary disenrollment rate (less than 2 percent).

Primary Care Physicians

There are two aspects to HMO-PA's effective use of primary care physicians. The first is the organizational and financial structure of HMO-PA's relationship with physicians, and the second is the quality of relations between physicians and the plan.

The model of the capitated, primary care gatekeeper works well for HMO-PA. Strict selection and recertification procedures are enforced by the physicians themselves. Once physicians have joined, and as long as they meet financial goals and do not cause patients to complain, they are not burdened with protocols, tight restrictions on referrals, precertification requirements, or other constraints on their autonomy. Physicians are also given opportunities to reduce medical costs. Provider relations staff endeavor to educate physicians about the availability of home care, early discharge programs, and other low-cost alternatives. The combination of a risk limited to 20 percent of capitation payments and the significant potential for sharing surpluses from the hospital and specialist pools helps make regulation of practice patterns unnecessary. The "win-win" situation created by this structure is enhanced by HMO-PA's ongoing efforts to meet primary care physicians' needs.

HMO-PA pays constant attention to its physicians, reminding one of an observation from *In Search of Excellence* on enhancing productivity through paying positive attention to people: "Management of mining companies that are good in exploration have scores of ways of paying attention to field geologists." The provider relations staff of HMO-PA assist physicians in a variety of ways, such as by training office managers and helping in the recruitment of new associate physicians. They also maintain open telephone lines for communication, make office visits, and regularly prepare newsletters to update physicians on HMO events and policies.

Prudent Purchasing of Medical Care

Prudent purchasing of hospital care and other medical services is critical to competitive pricing. HMO-PA has made a series of decisions about the structure and purchasing of care that have contained costs and transferred risk to providers. This, in turn, has enabled HMO-PA to price its services competitively and to successfully penetrate the market.

HMO-PA has secured favorable purchasing arrangements in two main ways: by using market clout to negotiate payment terms and levels and by developing innovative reimbursement mechanisms. It has negotiated all-inclusive hospital per diems that are comparable to rates paid by Blue Cross and lower than those paid by other HMOs in Philadelphia. It has also negotiated per case reimbursement with several hospitals as well as fixed rates for most ambulatory surgery procedures. The plan has capitated a broad array of services in addition to primary care: laboratory, podiatry, mental health, and outpatient radiology. Finally, HMO-PA is continually seeking new ways of relating to providers in order to control costs, reduce risk, and increase predictability of costs. The latest example is the full-risk capitation contract HMO-PA has signed with two teaching hospital staffs.

General Management

HMO-PA has mastered four key areas of management: marketing, provider relations, finance and administration, and human resources. Since the first two areas have been discussed earlier, this section focuses on finance-administration and human resources management.

An HMO must purchase or create effective, state-of-the-art systems for claims management, budget and rate setting, computerized information systems, and enrollment. These basic tools of the insurance business are not especially exciting, but they are indispensable; systems are constantly being improved to respond to enrollment growth and technological change.

HMO-PA employees are well motivated, express positive attitudes toward the company, and share a common business philosophy. While the company has developed programs and policies to build morale and motivate employees, it is difficult to separate the effects of these policies from the euphoria of success and rapid growth. The current rate of growth nationwide obviously creates both an exciting work environment and opportunities for career advancement. At the same time, HMO-PA has a major commitment to employee training, a system of incentive-based compensation with profit sharing, and a record of promotion from within. Personnel policies that repay employees for unused sick leave and an employee wellness program that rewards staff with a red HMO-PA sweatsuit for jogging on the company track are additional motivators. Finally, the authors of *In Search of Excellence* postulate that one of the most important motivating forces is personal attention from high-level managers. Thus, Len Abramson's penchant for "management by walking around" may be yet another contribution to what appears to be effective personnel management.

Many of the managers responsible for HMO-PA's success have moved into corporate-level positions at U. S. Healthcare. The top three people at U. S. Healthcare have been with HMO-PA since its inception, and the average tenure of the 11 most senior managers is 5½ years—a low rate of turnover for an organization founded in 1977. The executive management team is backed up by an echelon of middle managers who have for the most part risen from entry-level positions. This pattern of long tenure and promotion from within has resulted in a remarkably consistent corporate style. Difficult to characterize, this style or philosophy of management is market- and customer-oriented and emanates in large part from the personality and philosophy of the president.

Conclusions

The basic HMO-PA model, modified according to local opportunities and circumstances, has done well in terms of rapid growth and high profits both in the Philadelphia market and outside it. HMO-PA understands the niche it wants to occupy and is directed toward that objective. In selecting providers, for example, it does not try to be all things to all people. Obstetrician-gynecologists cannot be primary care physicians because they generally refer patients for problems other primary care physicians would handle. Not all the top hospitals are participating; if any hospital, even a highly desirable one, will not offer terms that are acceptable to HMO-PA, it is excluded from participation.

A market philosophy permeates many aspects of HMO-PA's operations. The modus operandi is to provide incentives rather than to regulate in order to achieve desired outcomes. Rigid utilization control systems are by and large avoided, but utilization data are monitored for underservice and overservice, which is defined as variations from the norm in either direction. A combination of the sentinel effect, financial incentives, and peer review accomplishes these ends. Inappropriately high levels of utilization (that is, above the budget targets) result in diminished compensation. Underservice or poor quality of care tends to generate consumer complaints, resulting in actions by HMO-PA to educate the individual physician.

Part IV
Lifeguard

16

Introduction

Lifeguard is a federally qualified, nonprofit, IPA-model HMO with headquarters in Campbell, California, which is just south of San Jose in Santa Clara County. The plan opened its doors in 1979 and now has 75,000 enrollees from four counties south and east of the San Francisco Bay, two-thirds of whom live in the San Jose area. It contracts with about 2,000 physicians, most of whom are in solo or small group practices, although four large multispecialty group practices also participate. In addition, Lifeguard has contractual arrangements with 14 hospitals.

Despite tough competition from Kaiser and 12 other HMOs, Lifeguard has continued to grow (see table 16.1). The plan is available to groups of 50 or more employees. Lifeguard currently has no Medicare or Medicaid beneficiaries, although it is applying for a Medicare risk contract.

The plan has also been successful financially. It broke even in 1981 and has remained in the black since, with a steadily increasing surplus. Last year the plan had revenues of nearly $33 million and reserves of $3,166,000.

In an effort to replicate Lifeguard's success elsewhere, key executives and board members in 1982 created IPA-USA, a for-profit management firm. This new venture is more than 90 percent owned by Lifeguard but has a separate board of directors. IPA-USA currently operates two physician-sponsored plans: the Health Plan of Mid-America in Kansas City, Missouri, and Best-care in Portland, Oregon.

Table 16.1
Lifeguard Membership
Growth

Year*	Members
1979	0
1980	7,793
1981	14,470
1982	24,920
1983	34,620
1984	48,040
1985	65,160†

* As of January.

† In August 1985, Lifeguard had
75,000 members.

This report is an account of some of the reasons for the success of Lifeguard. Chapter 17 characterizes the medical marketplace in which the plan operates. Chapter 18 presents an overview of the plan and addresses such topics as the plan's history, relations with physicians and hospitals, quality assurance and utilization review, marketing, consumer relations, and organizational culture and management philosophy. Finally, the factors that appear to account for the plan's success are summarized in chapter 19.

17

The Market

The demographic and economic characteristics of Lifeguard's service area are somewhat favorable for HMO development, but the medical marketplace is reasonably disciplined and highly competitive. The plan serves a population that is well educated, affluent, and growing but also characterized by low hospital utilization rates and lower than average per capita hospital expenses. This decreases the opportunities for HMOs to realize savings and, together with the influx of HMOs and PPOs, has created a highly competitive health plan environment.

This chapter presents data by county or by metropolitan statistical area, depending on which is available. Lifeguard's four-county service area falls into three MSAs—San Jose, Oakland, and Vallejo-Fairfield-Napa—but Lifeguard does not serve all of the territory encompassed by these MSAs.

Demographic and Economic Characteristics

Lifeguard originated in Santa Clara County and then expanded into Alameda, Contra Costa, and Solano counties. Santa Clara County contains Silicon Valley, the area between Palo Alto and San Jose in which hundreds of electronics companies are concentrated; most of these companies are self-insured. The cities of Oakland and Berkeley are in Alameda County. Contra Costa and Solano counties encompass the less urban areas between Oakland and Sacramento.

This service area has 3.3 million people and is growing. Santa Clara County, with 1.3 million people, grew by almost 22 percent between 1970 and 1980 (see table 17.1). Only Alameda County, with an increase of 3 percent, grew more slowly than the national average of 11 percent during the decade. Another positive feature from the standpoint of HMO development is the age of the service area population, which is younger than the U.S. average. Only 7 percent of Santa Clara County's residents are 65 or over, in contrast to the national average of almost 12 percent. The only county approaching the national age distribution is Alameda, with 11 percent of the population over age 65.[1]

One of the most striking characteristics of the service area is the affluence of its residents. All four counties have median incomes considerably higher than the U.S. median of $19,917. The highest median income—$26,659, more than a third above the national norm—is in Santa Clara. The population is also well educated. Three of the four counties have well above average levels of educational attainment for secondary schooling, while Solano is at the national norm, with about 67 percent of its residents having completed at least 12 years of school. In Contra Costa County, with the best educated population, 82 percent of residents have attained this level of education (see table 17.1).

Given these data, it is not surprising that all four counties have low rates of poverty and unemployment. The percentage of the population below the poverty level ranges from 7 in Santa Clara County to 11 in Alameda County, compared to a national average of more than 12 percent. Unemployment rates fluctuate but generally run below the national average in all counties except Solano; in January 1985, unemployment was about 5 percent in Santa Clara, 7 percent in Contra Costa and Alameda, and 9 percent in Solano, compared to the national figure of 8 percent.

Medical Cost and Supply Factors

The medical market in California is a disciplined one, reflecting perhaps the long-standing experience with both Kaiser and the foundations for medical care as well as the prevalence of prepayment. California has a higher percentage of its population enrolled in HMOs (22 percent) than any other state, and HMO penetration in the San Francisco Bay Area approaches 40 percent. Hospital utilization rates on the West Coast have traditionally been among the lowest in the nation. Hospital utilization and ex-

Table 17.1

Population and Socioeconomic Characteristics of the Lifeguard Service Area

County	1980 Population	Change Since 1970 (%)	Over Age 65, 1983 (%)	Median Family Income, 1979 ($)	Below Poverty Level, 1979 (%)	Unemployment Rate, January 1985 (%)	High School Graduates, 1983 (%)
Alameda	1,105,000	+ 3.2	11.3	22,863	11.3	7.3	76.0
Contra Costa	656,400	+18.0	7.6	26,510	7.6	6.7	81.7
Santa Clara	1,295,000	+21.6	7.1	26,659	7.1	5.1	79.5
Solano	235,200	+36.8	9.4	21,606	9.4	9.4	66.5
Total	3,292,000	—	—	—	—	—	—
U.S. Average	—	11.4	11.7	19,917	12.4	8.0	66.5

Source: U.S. Department of Commerce, Bureau of the Census, *County and City Data Book—1983* (Washington, D.C.: Government Printing Office, 1983); U.S. Department of Labor, Bureau of Labor Statistics, personal communication.

penses per capita in Lifeguard's service area are below the state
and national averages as well.

In 1983, hospital expenses per capita ranged from $432 in the
Vallejo-Fairfield-Napa MSA to $508 in the Oakland MSA, com-
pared to a national MSA average of $560. In the San Jose MSA,
where the bulk of Lifeguard enrollees live, hospital expenses averaged $502 per capita.[2]

Utilization data are especially striking (see table 17.2). By
every measure of hospital utilization, the counties in Lifeguard's
service area are below national norms. Data are available only for
Santa Clara County and for Alameda and Contra Costa counties
combined; thus in 1983

— Hospital days per thousand persons were some 40 percent
  below the U.S. average.

— Admissions per thousand persons were about 25 percent
  lower.

— The average length of stay was 5.9 days in Santa Clara
  County and 6.2 in Alameda–Contra Costa, compared with
  7.6 for the entire United States.

— The hospital occupancy rate was 69 percent in all three
  counties, compared to 74 percent nationwide, despite a
  low supply of beds relative to the nation as a whole.

Supply of hospital beds is low, reflecting the pattern of low
utilization. The average number of beds per thousand persons is
2.8 in Santa Clara County and 3.0 in Alameda–Contra Costa, well
below the national average of 4.5. In contrast to the low bed supply, there are more physicians per capita than the U.S. average in
all counties but Solano. In Santa Clara county, Lifeguard's center
of operations, there are 2.9 M.D.'s per thousand persons, compared to 2.1 per thousand nationally. A generous supply of physicians is generally construed as helpful to HMO development.

Taken together, these data indicate that there is relatively
little fat in the health care delivery system in and around Santa
Clara County, at least as measured by traditional rules of thumb.

The Health Insurance Market

The health insurance market is highly competitive throughout
Lifeguard's service area. Health maintenance organizations are
not competing against indemnity plans as much as against other
HMOs, as the very low utilization data suggest.

Table 17.2

Medical Supply and Utilization Factors in the Lifeguard Service Area, 1983

County	M.D.'s per 1,000 Persons*	Inpatient Days per 1,000 Persons	Admissions per 1,000 Persons	Hospital Beds per 1,000 Persons	Average Length of Stay (Days)	Occupancy Rate (%)
Alameda/ Contra Costa	2.6	743	121	3.0	6.2	69
Santa Clara	2.9	697	119	2.8	5.9	69
Solano	1.5	N.A.	N.A.	N.A.	N.A.	N.A.
United States	2.1	1,206	159	4.5	7.6	74

Sources: American Hospital Association, *Hospital Statistics* (Chicago: AHA, 1984); American Medical Association, personal communication; U.S. Department of Commerce, Bureau of the Census, *Statistical Abstract of the United States, 1985* (Washington, D.C.: Government Printing Office, 1984).

* As of 1981.

N.A. indicates data are not available.

Even so, the Blues are viewed as significant competitors. Blue Shield and Blue Cross are separate plans in California; unlike elsewhere, both cover hospital and physician services and compete against each other. The plans have achieved relatively low penetration of the market. Other non-HMO competition includes proprietary hospital chains that are entering the health insurance business and growing numbers of self-insured employers. Many self-insured employers are raising deductibles and reducing benefits without increasing their contributions, making it more difficult for Lifeguard and other HMOs to attract enrollees.

As of December 1984, there were a dozen HMOs, serving one or more counties in Lifeguard's service area (see table 17.3). Lifeguard's major competitors at present are Kaiser, TakeCare (the Blue Cross HMO), Maxicare, IPM Health Plan, Heals, and Foundation Health Plan. Other established plans, such as Bay Pacific, operate in nearby San Mateo and San Francisco counties; they make expansion more difficult for Lifeguard and have moved into Lifeguard's territory.

This mature market does not seem to deter new entrants, however, and competition is intensifying. Major national HMO firms and hospital systems probably pose the greatest threat, and several PPOs are under development. The plan is less concerned about competition from PPOs; in the view of Dorothy Emerson, executive vice president of Lifeguard, "the PPO is just a dressed-up insurance policy." The types of changes occurring in Lifeguard's market are summarized below.

— Maxicare, the third largest and one of the fastest growing investor-owned HMO chains in the United States, expanded to Northern California in 1984. Although it has not made much headway to date, Maxicare is a potentially formidable competitor.

— Prudent Buyer, a Blue Cross PPO, has been particularly aggressive in attempts to expand its market share in recent months.

— Pacificare, the Los Angeles–based HMO, recently went public and is considering expansion into Northern California.

— National Medical Enterprises, a proprietary hospital chain, is reportedly starting a prepaid plan in the San Francisco area.

Many plans moving into Lifeguard territory have major financial reserves, and Lifeguard is concerned that they could afford to run at a loss for a significant period of time.

There is still room to increase overall HMO penetration in Lifeguard's service area, but it is quite possible that not all of these competitors will survive. Lifeguard's market penetration ranges from 0.2 to 4 percent in the four counties it serves, while overall HMO penetration in those counties exceeds 40 percent.

Notes

1. While an aged population has been considered less desirable for HMOs due to both higher costs of care for older people and the inability to enroll Medicare beneficiaries on an at-risk basis, this may be changing as new provisions for enrolling Medicare beneficiaries in HMOs are implemented.

2. American Hospital Association, *Hospital Statistics* (Chicago: AHA, 1984).

Table 17.3

HMOs in the Lifeguard Service Area

Plan	Year Formed	Model	Members	
			June 1981	December 1984
Lifeguard HMO Campbell	1979	IPA	18,000	65,000
Kaiser Permanente (Northern California) Oakland	1945	Group	1,723,200	1,926,000
Maxicare (Northern and Southern California)* Hawthorne	1973	Network	110,000	207,000
Foundation Health Plan Sacramento	1978	IPA	39,300	105,000
TakeCare Corporation Oakland	1978	Network	31,400	103,000
Health Plan of America Oakland	1980	IPA	450	27,300
HealthAmerica Rockridge Albany	1974	Network	13,100	27,000
Heals-Personal Care Physicians Health Emeryville	1981	IPA	0	25,900

Table 17.3—continued

HMOs in the Lifeguard Service Area

Plan	Year Formed	Model	Members	
			June 1981	December 1984
IPM Health Plan Vallejo	1979	Network	5,000	16,300
French Hospital Health Plan San Francisco	1851	Staff	4,800	13,000
Children's Hospital Health Plan San Francisco	1975	IPA	10,600	11,100
Contra Costa Health Plan Martinez	1974	Staff	5,700	11,100

Source: Modified from InterStudy, *National HMO Census—1981* (Excelsior, Minn.: InterStudy, 1981) and *National HMO Census—1984* (Excelsior, Minn.: InterStudy, 1985).

* Approximately 1 percent of these members are in Northern California.

18

Overview

Lifeguard is a nonprofit IPA-model HMO that evolved out of the Foundation for Medical Care of the Santa Clara County Medical Society. The foundation was created in 1959 and was the first countywide attempt by fee-for-service physicians to conduct peer review. The foundation was not financially at risk, but physicians did agree to offer their services on a discounted basis to insurers who contracted with the foundation. In that regard, it was similar to some of the PPOs of today. Insurers were contractually required to cover ambulatory care and provide equal benefits for dependents. Dorothy Emerson was the foundation's first employee. Foreshadowing her later accomplishments at Lifeguard, she was in charge of establishing review systems to conduct quality and utilization audits. The foundation worked with various insurance carriers and ultimately enrolled about 125,000 people.

In 1973, Emerson and Robert Burnett, M.D., now president of Lifeguard, collaborated on a project sponsored jointly by the foundation and Blue Cross, called Emcare. Like an HMO, Emcare offered a comprehensive benefits package; however, the foundation did not accept risk (Blue Cross did). The project was terminated in 1975, largely because the foundation and Blue Cross had differing goals.

The process of planning Lifeguard started at this time. Burnett, then president of the Santa Clara Medical Society, and Emerson, with over 15 years' experience in analyzing local physician practice patterns, had close ties to the medical community and were personally acquainted with many area physicians and hospitals. They modeled Lifeguard on an IPA in Sacramento that also had foundation origins.

Applications for membership were circulated to local physicians through the medical society. About 450 of the 1,200 medical society members signed up with Lifeguard initially. Dorothy Emerson believes that primary care physicians joined because plan enrollees were being offered first-dollar coverage for the first time. Specialists followed, to preserve their referral sources. Physicians were required to accept a fee schedule and a 15 percent risk retention; they were also assessed a $100 membership fee. Much of the early operating capital came from the providers: each of the original four participating hospitals paid $100,000 to join. In addition, a federal loan for $1.2 million was obtained in 1979.

Despite the founders' years of experience in managing health care, their familiarity with Santa Clara County, and a medical community that was reasonably receptive to their endeavor, there were problems to overcome. One of the hardest tasks was to educate physicians about utilization. A favorite method of education, initiated by Emerson, was sending a copy of the hospital bill to every physician who had worked on a case (surgeon, assistant surgeon, anesthesiologist, and so on). Lifeguard only recently stopped circulating hospital bills. The rigorous utilization review systems now in operation are unique to Lifeguard and represent an evolution from earlier efforts at Emcare and the foundation.

Lifeguard is an open-panel HMO and affords members a wide choice of delivery sites for medical care. The plan contracts with about 2,000 physicians and pays them according to a fee schedule. It also has arrangements with 14 hospitals and other specialized providers, such as surgicenters. Lifeguard members are required to choose a personal physician from among a list of primary care physicians that includes family practitioners, internists, pediatricians, and obstetrician-gynecologists. The primary care physician serves as a case manager and must authorize all referrals for specialty care. It is frequently possible for new Lifeguard members to continue seeing their private physician, if he or she is a Lifeguard provider. In addition to the cost control resulting from a gatekeeper physician, all inpatient care and certain other services and procedures must be explicitly authorized by the plan. Unless authorized, care is not covered by the plan, and patients, who are not held harmless, may be liable for the charges.

Lifeguard offers a single package of basic benefits, with optional riders for drug and vision care. The plan covers ambulatory services with certain restrictions (for example, one health evaluation per year after age 2) and provides unlimited acute-care hospitalization when authorized. Inpatient psychotherapy for the acute phase of a mental condition (such as alcohol detoxification but not rehabilitation) is covered for up to 30 days per year. Emergency care is paid for whether in or out of Lifeguard's service area, although the plan's literature stresses that these services will be reimbursed only if they were medically necessary. Skilled nursing facility, home health, and ambulance services are covered when medically necessary. In general, the benefits package is slightly more restrictive than that of many other HMOs, although Lifeguard does cover durable medical equipment in part, unlike many other HMOs.

The plan has extensive (for an HMO) cost-sharing features, both in the form of flat copayments and coinsurance. The major provisions for cost sharing include

— Copayments for health evaluations that vary by age: 2–6, $5 per visit; 7–17, $10 per visit; 18 and over, $25 per visit

— Routine office visit, $3

— Eye examination and refraction (under age 18 only, no more than one per year), $10

— Outpatient psychotherapy, 50 percent of charges per visit (up to $20)

— Emergency room (when authorized) and urgent after-hours visit, $15

— Infertility studies, 50 percent of charges

— Durable medical equipment (when prescribed), 50 percent of charges

— Varying copayments for prescription drugs and vision care, depending on contract

Relations With Providers

One lasting effect of Lifeguard's foundation origins is its relations with physicians and hospitals. Lifeguard views itself as an insurer, serving as broker between physicians and patients. It does not seek to impose any particular culture or set of values upon member physicians, other than a mandate to share responsibility for peer review. Lifeguard's priority in provider relations is prompt payment for all services rendered in accordance with the plan's benefit package and utilization standards.

Physicians

Most of Lifeguard's physicians are in solo or small partnership practice, although the plan also has relations with four sizable groups, including the prestigious Palo Alto Medical Foundation and Sunnyvale Medical Clinic. Lifeguard originally created three IPAs in its service area in order to be able to contract for physician services. When subsequent changes in California law and federal qualification requirements allowed HMOs to contract directly with individual physicians, Lifeguard stopped contracting with IPAs, largely because plan administrators believe that dealing with IPAs as entities tends to introduce unnecessary conflict. Instead, Lifeguard now contracts directly with individual physicians.

Efforts to recruit physicians are minimal. Physicians abound in the service area, and the plan has as many as it requires. Some two-thirds of Lifeguard's physicians are in Santa Clara County, the location of corporate headquarters. Specialists, relative to need, are more plentiful than primary care physicians. Lifeguard does not require that physicians enter into an exclusive relationship with the plan; in fact, it encourages them to participate in other health plans so that Lifeguard is not their primary source of revenue.

The selection process is not stringent. Essentially, all physicians who meet the three basic criteria are accepted: (1) they must be members in good standing, or eligible for membership, in the medical society; (2) they must have privileges at a participating hospital; and (3) they must carry adequate malpractice insurance. Membership in the medical society is viewed as a proxy for other standards. Applications from physicians are no longer being accepted. Before membership was closed, physicians paid a $1,000 fee to join and waited 18 months before starting to see Lifeguard patients. In Lifeguard's early days, the fee was $100 and there was no waiting period.

The quality of care delivered by participating physicians is assessed primarily by comparing utilization patterns with Lifeguard's standards for reasonable use of services. (The quality assurance and utilization review systems are described in detail below.) No physician has ever been asked to leave, although several have been placed "on review" for inappropriate practice patterns; in such cases, all referrals, tests, and procedures ordered by the physician are scrutinized. Whenever Lifeguard has initiated steps to remove a physician—perhaps a dozen times in eight years— that physician has changed the behavior in question.

Compensation is on a fee-for-service basis, using a schedule that draws heavily on the California Relative Value Scale. Starting with the scale, Lifeguard's top managers added procedures and adapted some codes. The major philosophical change was a modest shift in conversion factors to reward time spent with the patient. The effect is to reimburse procedures (mostly surgical) at relatively lower levels than office visits. In general, Lifeguard pays fees that are comparable to the community standard for medicine (perhaps 10 percent less) and slightly lower for surgery (about 15 percent less).

Fifteen percent of physicians' fees (10 percent for physicians who have been with the plan for a long time) is withheld to cover any HMO deficit. Certain other providers (for example, some hospitals) also contribute to the risk pool. Lifeguard expects to return these funds to the physicians and other contributors at six-month intervals, and so far it always has. The HMO is at risk for losses beyond this 15 percent withholding, and it keeps any surplus. Physicians are not at risk for hospital budget deficits, nor do they share in any surpluses.

Hospitals and Other Providers

Lifeguard contracts with 13 community hospitals and Stanford Hospital, a tertiary care teaching facility. Terms of payment vary by hospital. The four original hospitals, each of which paid $100,000 to join in 1977, receive their full billed charges, whereas hospitals admitted more recently are typically paid on a per diem basis. A few hospitals are subject to a 15 percent risk withholding from billed charges; these funds become part of the risk pool described above, and distribution is based on the overall performance of the plan, not that of the individual hospital.

Lifeguard wanted Stanford to participate largely because it wanted to encourage Palo Alto Medical Clinic physicians to join. The Palo Alto Medical Clinic is a large multispecialty group in Santa Clara County whose members typically practice at nearby

Stanford Hospital. Lifeguard does not attempt to market its affiliation with Stanford and for cost reasons does not permit use of Stanford Children's Hospital or the Stanford outpatient clinics.

Lifeguard intends to add a few more hospitals, particularly in the vicinity of Stanford Hospital. Stanford Hospital is expensive, even with the modest discounts that have been negotiated, and the plan would like to divert nontertiary admissions away from it. Overall, however, Lifeguard does not believe that costs vary significantly among its major participating hospitals, and selection has typically been based on the preferences and admitting practices of Lifeguard physicians. The plan has never explicitly encouraged admission to one hospital over another, due to the small cost differentials among them and the plan's desire not to interfere with physician autonomy. One Lifeguard executive suggested that this could change as the environment becomes more competitive.

Lifeguard contracts with two surgicenters and is talking to others. The plan typically obtains discounts from standard rates, with the level of discount varying by diagnosis. In addition, several member hospitals have freestanding surgical centers that plan physicians may use.

Lifeguard has no special arrangements with skilled nursing facilities or home health agencies. It has no difficulty getting beds in skilled nursing facilities because it pays full charges. It uses the Visiting Nurses Association exclusively for home care but has thus far had little need for these services. The plan has no relations with particular pharmacies; members with drug benefits may use any retail pharmacy and file claims for reimbursement.

Quality Assurance and Utilization Review

Quality assurance and utilization review at Lifeguard are combined into one process. Concerns about quality of care are frequently raised in the course of utilization review and are addressed by a committee charged with monitoring both quality and utilization.

The hospital and ambulatory review systems are especially impressive. The need for capable utilization review systems for both inpatient and outpatient services is pronounced in such an HMO, where provider reimbursement is on a fee-for-service basis and risk sharing is collective rather than individual. The preadmission and concurrent reviews of hospital care are handled over the telephone by a staff of nurses, while ambulatory review is conducted through both automated and manual examination of claims.

The three sections below describe quality assurance at Lifeguard, the Certified Hospital Admission Program for preadmission and concurrent review of inpatient care and selected other services, and methods of ambulatory review. The controls for inpatient and ambulatory care operate independently of one another and therefore are discussed separately.

Quality Assurance

Primary responsibility for supervising quality assurance and utilization review rests with the Medical Quality Utilization Assurance Committee, which is comprised of about 20 Lifeguard physicians selected by the president and the executive vice president. Members are always primary care physicians who do not depend on referrals, and they are paid for their time. Specialty committees of Lifeguard physicians (pediatricians, surgeons, and so on) are on call as consultants to the committee.

At its monthly meetings, the committee addresses whatever issues have arisen; typically, these include

— Establishment of new reimbursement or medical policies
— Review of unusual requests for authorization, such as admission to a nonparticipating facility or permission to conduct special or experimental procedures
— Review of physician responses to letters from claims analysts questioning their utilization patterns
— Review of quality of care issues, particularly in reference to the management of individual cases or in response to consumer complaints

Quality of care issues may be raised in several ways: by physician advisers to the Certified Hospital Admissions Program, through review of outpatient or inpatient claims, and through the consumer relations department. The role of physician advisers in the hospital admissions process is described below; at their quarterly meetings, they review all hospital admissions for the previous three months. Lifeguard has an outstanding claims review process that is particularly adept at spotting overutilization, which in itself can indicate poor care. In addition, inappropriate

Table 18.1

Lifeguard Hospital
Utilization

Year	Inpatient Days per 1,000 Members*
1980	350
1981	364
1982	286
1983	274
1984	275
1985†	272

* Excludes newborns.
† Through June.

use of services, such as a series of laboratory tests performed without an accompanying physical examination, can also result in the detection of inadequate care. Finally, complaints from members can highlight problems with particular providers.

While there is no formal mechanism for identifying underservice beyond that described above, Lifeguard's management believes two other features of the plan improve quality of care and protect against underservice. First, paying physicians on a fee-for-service basis and not putting them at risk as individuals promotes quality because it creates no incentive to underserve. Second, Lifeguard's insistence that each member use one primary care physician is a mechanism for ensuring continuity and accountability, both of which are thought to be correlated with high-quality care.

Certified Hospital Admission Program

The Certified Hospital Admission Program (CHAP) combines pre-admission and concurrent, or length-of-stay, review. It is a major contributor to Lifeguard's low hospital utilization (see table 18.1). Lifeguard had 274 inpatient days per thousand members in 1983, compared to the Santa Clara County average of 697. As an example of its impact, the CHAP program is credited with reducing Lifeguard's average length of stay from two days to one day for tonsillectomies and from three days to just under two days for normal deliveries of babies.

Lifeguard requires that all elective hospital admissions be authorized in advance. In the case of an emergency admission, CHAP must be notified within 48 hours so that a nurse can authorize the admission and monitor the patient's condition. The usual authorization process for hospital care has five steps.

— For nonemergency cases, the Lifeguard physician notifies CHAP nurses of an impending admission at least 24 hours in advance.

— A CHAP nurse approves the admission and assigns a tentative length of stay. The nurse completes a form recording patient eligibility status, availability of other insurance for coordination of benefits, hospital name, admitting diagnosis, proposed surgery or procedure, a brief history, names of primary care and admitting physicians, and the proposed length of stay. This form is referred to throughout the patient's hospital stay.

— At the time of admission, the hospital calls a CHAP nurse to obtain a certifiction number, which the hospital knows is necessary for its claim to be paid. Information on the CHAP form is verified.

— Utilization review nurses, employed by the hospital, review Lifeguard patients daily and telephone a report to the CHAP nurses. Each case is discussed briefly, and the CHAP nurse records the condition of the patient on his or her form.

— As soon as a patient appears to be making progress, the CHAP nurse begins to anticipate discharge. If a patient is recovering at a faster rate than predicted, the CHAP nurse may call the attending physician and ask about early discharge. If the length of stay is extended, the nurse may ask the physician about the possibility of home care.

All three CHAP nurses (two registered nurses and one licensed practical nurse) have clinical experience, and they try to make determinations on a case-by-case basis. Formal length-of-stay norms have not been adopted, although decisions do reflect the community standard, insurance company policies, and Medicare guidelines. In addition, several policies have been formulated, among them the following:

— Evening and weekend admissions are generally not permitted; physicians are encouraged to have laboratory work performed on an outpatient basis or early in the morning on the day of surgery.

— For certain diagnoses, home care is commonly suggested as an alternative (for example, home traction for back problems).

— Hysterectomies for women under age 35 require a second opinion before they can be authorized (Lifeguard selects the physician and pays for the consultant).

— Certain procedures should generally be performed on an outpatient basis, barring extenuating circumstances; the list is a fairly standard one and includes, for example, arthroscopy, adenoidectomy, and cataract surgery.

— Other procedures (for example, hernia repair) are often performed on an outpatient basis, at the physician's discretion; the CHAP nurse may ask the physician if this is an option in a particular case.

When new surgeries or procedures arise, groups of specialists participating in Lifeguard are convened to recommend policy for coverage and guidelines for authorization.

Other institutional care, such as admission to a skilled nursing facility, must be authorized in the same way. Some inpatient procedures require authorization themselves, in addition to the authorization to admit. A number of outpatient procedures and services (for example, home health care, physical therapy) must also be authorized through CHAP.

When requests for authorization fall outside standard policies, they are assigned to a Lifeguard physician adviser, who reviews the proposed admission and, if approved, assigns a length of stay. Two physician advisers cover each participating hospital. They are respected specialists in private practice who perform the procedures they are reviewing. CHAP nurses call on them an average of once or twice a month.

Certain outpatient and inpatient procedures require written rather than telephone authorization, for example, amniocentesis, lithotripsy, and magnetic resonance imaging. In these cases, the referring physician calls a CHAP nurse to request a letter of authorization, which the patient presents at the time of service. The provider then submits this letter with a bill for payment.

Beyond the formal structure described are the training and skill of the CHAP nurses and their respected leader, Tracy Metz, R.N., vice president of health care delivery. For concurrent review, CHAP relies on utilization review nurses employed by the individual hospitals. Lifeguard has developed good relationships with these key people, which the CHAP staff maintain. As a result, the plan constantly receives information about its patients by telephone. The concurrent review process requires much day-to-day management yet is extremely efficient.

In addition to daily monitoring of hospitalized members, the CHAP department produces monthly utilization reports. These summarize hospital days used per 1,000 members by service (medicine, surgery, psychiatry, obstetrics, pediatrics), provide data on average length of stay and cost per day by hospital, and itemize the number of premature births and their associated costs.

Ambulatory Review

The ambulatory review process is automated. This is especially appropriate for an HMO such as Lifeguard because (1) the plan pays for ambulatory services on a fee-for-service basis; (2) it has claims data; and (3) it lacks any opportunity to observe practice patterns and educate physicians in an informal or collegial way, as group- or staff-model HMOs commonly do.

Lifeguard's ambulatory review depends on an efficient claims system. The typical turnaround time (between receiving and paying a claim) is three to five days. Rapid claims processing is important for two reasons:

— Claims must be entered into the system promptly in order for the records to be complete. When new incoming claims are reviewed against an incomplete record, inappropriate payments or incorrect denials can result.

— Prompt payment assures good provider relations.

The plan has the capacity to process claims (both inpatient and outpatient) the day they are received or the following day, and checks are drawn weekly. Some 10 computer input operators enter claims. If there is insufficient terminal capacity, claims are processed manually and data entered into the computer later. (About 10 percent of claims are processed manually.) At the time of data entry, claims representing the following are automatically set aside for review:

— A procedure for which a relative value has not been established

— A procedure not in the coding manual

— Multiple surgical procedures on the same patient

These claims are sent to physicians, who are paid $25 per claim, to establish units for payment. In addition, claims may be held for coordination of benefits if the enrollee has duplicate coverage through another plan. Information for coordinating benefits is acquired through both the eligibility and the claims process, and enrollees are resurveyed periodically.

Once the data are entered into the system, Lifeguard's ambulatory review has two main components, the individual claim screen and retrospective utilization review. This structure reflects Dorothy Emerson's view that the plan cannot do profiling or peer review if there are "parts of claims sitting on everyone's desk."

Individual Claim Screen. The individual claim screen, which Lifeguards calls "broad screen," is a way of identifying claims that should not be paid until they are investigated further. The term is used by the plan in two different ways. Broadly, it reflects Lifeguard's philosophy that some maximum amount of diagnostic or therapeutic procedures should be allowed without being questioned, that is, without considering the diagnosis or other special circumstances. Specifically, it refers to particular limits, beyond which a claim is held for review. For example, there is a screen for claims from multiple physicians for one patient with the same diagnosis, for potentially excessive diagnostic testing, and so forth (see table 18.2).

The patient profile is at the center of the individual claim screen system. This profile is generated from claims data accumulated over the previous 18 months. It includes all outpatient physician services, ancillary services, and drugs, with diagnoses and providers identified. Finally, it is linked to each member's original application, which has information on eligibility and coordination of benefits.

The process for screening individual claims is as follows:

— When a claim is entered into the system, it is evaluated as part of the existing patient profile and either passes or fails the screen. If it passes, the claim is paid.

— If the claim fails the screen, the claims analyst can make a determination to pay under certain circumstances (for

Table 18.2

Examples of Individual Claim Screen Limits

Physician Visits
- More than one health evaluation per year
- Visits to more than one physician for the same or similar diagnoses
- Use of more than one primary care physician in one year
- More than one visit per week, two visits per month, three visits per quarter, or four visits per year

Ancillary Services
- More than four urinalyses per quarter
- More than one hemoglobin test per year
- More than two Pap smears per year

Cost
- More than $200 in outpatient pharmacy costs in six months
- Procedure bill in excess of $500

Other
- More than one emergency visit per quarter
- Procedure performed on wrong sex
- Procedure performed more than once (for example, two hysterectomies)

example, if the amount is less than $500); otherwise, it is forwarded for review.

— Review entails sending a copy of the claim and the patient profile to a Lifeguard physician for his or her opinion of the treatment, given the diagnosis.

— If the reviewing physician is unwilling to make a decision, the information is sent to additional reviewing physicians. If the issue still cannot be resolved, a panel of physicians is convened to meet with the physician who submitted the claim in order to reach a decision.

Some 2,000 to 3,000 claims are received each day. About 25 percent of them do not pass the individual claim screen; of these, 60 percent are overriden by the claims analysts. Thus about 10 percent of all claims are subjected to physician review.

Retrospective Review. For retrospective review, all cases in which the individual claim screen limits (see table 18.2) were exceeded are printed out every two weeks. When patterns of apparent overutilization appear, even if claims were overriden by analysts and paid, standard letters are sent to physicians highlighting the problem and asking them whether the overuse was inadvertent on their part or the fault of the patient. Repeated incidents involving the same physician will be identified from the physician profile (see table 18.3), and further action may be taken.

Further action could entail a more direct letter, perhaps from the medical director, or an invitation to the physician to present his or her position before a panel of Lifeguard physician peers. In the extreme, a physician will be placed "on review," and all his or her claims will be checked for appropriateness for a period of time. However, the goal is to change behavior, not to deny payment. This is one reason bills are often paid yet accompanied by a letter questioning the necessity or appropriateness of services rendered.

Marketing

Lifeguard concentrates its marketing efforts on employers who do not currently offer HMOs. Few employers are willing to offer more than the minimum of two HMOs (one IPA and one closed-panel model) mandated by federal law. The plan will occasionally approach very large employers, mostly those with more than 1,000 employees, and try to "dislodge" the existing IPA. However, it will not pursue this strategy if it does not receive a favorable reception during the first one or two calls. Lifeguard is also increasingly concerned that, with HMO growth in the area, it could be displaced by other IPAs employing a similar strategy.

Many firms throughout the service area have restrictive benefits, often through self-insured plans, a situation that is not conducive to HMO enrollment. However, the nature of the competition differs by county. Santa Clara and Alameda counties have had high HMO penetration for some time, mostly as a result of Kaiser, and many have had dealings with IPAs. As a result, employers in those counties understand IPAs. In contrast, employers in Contra Costa and Solano counties are less familiar with IPAs.

The entire service area is witnessing heightened competition, and Lifeguard is concerned that the new HMOs have deeper pockets than it does, particularly those that are for-profit or insurer-based or both and can afford to operate at a loss if necessary. On the other hand, one person commented that, with the large number of physician members that Lifeguard has signed up, "We have the product, and they don't."

Lifeguard's marketing strategy is purposely conservative and somewhat narrowly focused. The plan markets mostly to groups with more than 100 employees and generally will not cover

Table 18.3

Reports Generated by the Ambulatory Review System

Patient Profiles
All physician, hospital, and ancillary services for an 18-month period, by provider
- Provider name and identification number
- Diagnosis (CRVS and ICDA codes)
- Total amount billed
- Patient copayment
- Lifeguard benefit amount
- COB deductions
- Risk retention amount (15%)
- Net amount paid

Physician Profiles
Avaiable for individual physicians and by specialty
- Type of service (drugs, visits, procedures, and so on)
- Number of services
- Plan benefit
- Services per patient by age and sex
- Cost per service by procedure (CRVS)
- Cost per patient by procedure (CRVS)
- Cost per diagnosis (ICDA code)

Age and Sex Profiles
Available for individual physicians and in the aggregate, by age and sex
- Number of services
- Number of patients
- Plan benefit
- Cost per patient

Diagnostic Profiles
Using ICDA diagnostic code, lists patients with a given diagnosis seen by each physician (includes inpatient physician care but not hospital charges)
- Patient name and date of service
- Total amount billed
- Patient copayment
- Plan benefit
- Other deductions (COB)
- Risk retention (15%)
- Net amount paid

Referring Physician Profile
Lists physician (or other agent, such as laboratory or hospital) receiving the referral, including patient services
- Patient name
- CRVS diagnostic code
- Plan benefit
- Risk retention
- Amount paid

Table 18.3—continued

Reports Generated by the Ambulatory Review System

Summary of Referring Physician Profile
For each physician, lists all referrals made and all referral services
covered by Lifeguard

- Referred physician services
- Referred laboratory services
- Referred X-ray services
- Prescription drugs
- Total outpatient benefits
- Total inpatient benefits

Comparison of Office Cost and Medical Referral Cost
Produced every six months for individual physicians and specialties

- Physician name
- Total number of Lifeguard patients
- Physician's charges and amount paid
- Physician's referral costs
- Total average cost per patient (cost of this physician plus referral
  costs)

---

groups with fewer than 50 employees. All of Lifeguard's 10 largest
employer groups are private firms rather than government agencies, which distinguishes the plan from many other HMOs. It
recently signed a contract with the Federal Employee Health Benefits Program but is wary of too large a federal enrollment. Individual coverage is offered only as a conversion from group coverage, and the option to convert is not actively promoted. The plan
has signed up only four Taft-Hartley trust funds, although it is increasing its marketing efforts to unions. The plan does not have
Medicaid enrollment but is seriously investigating whether to enter into a risk contract with Medicare.

The plan, like most others, declines to enroll certain groups
through its underwriting practices. Between 20 and 30 percent of
prospects are not pursued. Firms with high premium differentials
compared to the indemnity plan, such as most retail outlets, are
typically avoided, because enrollments would probably be low
and Lifeguard would be adversely selected against. Firms with
high turnover are also avoided, as are salespeople paid on commission, because premiums cannot be collected through payroll
deduction.

Lifeguard particularly seeks to attract enrollees away from
other HMOs, as opposed to indemnity plans. Indeed, within em-

ployer groups, about half of new enrollees were previously members of other HMOs, and some 80 percent of them were enrolled in Kaiser. Families who switch out of Kaiser face a $13 to $14 monthly premium increase. The advantages of Lifeguard that are stressed in presentations to prospective enrollees include the following:

— Access to more than 2,000 practicing physicians (thus, a new enrollee not currently enrolled in an HMO may be able to retain his or her doctor)

— Access to a personal physician who is on call 24 hours a day

— Comprehensiveness of coverage, including ambulatory care

— Prevention ("Lifeguard keeps you well")

— The absence of claims forms

— Easy access to a consumer relations department

Senior executives of Lifeguard believe that a significant factor in the plan's success is that it offers a single product which is easily understood by enrollees and providers alike.

The hospital network is not emphasized in marketing. Also, physicians are not expected to assist in marketing; plan management believes that adverse selection would occur were they to seek to enroll their own patients.

The marketing function is performed by a staff of 13, including secretarial and clerical personnel who help with correspondence and follow-up telephone calls. The director of marketing has two managers, one responsible for Santa Clara County and part of Alameda County, and the other for the expansion territories in Contra Costa and Solano counties. New staff receive mostly on-the-job, rather than formal classroom, training. However, they do role-play oral presentations, which are videotaped and critiqued by experienced marketing representatives. Training covers the benefit package, the nature of the plan, the open enrollment process, how to perform comparisons of benefits, how to approach employers, and so forth.

The marketing staff are paid straight salaries. Commissions and bonuses have not been instituted, in order to minimize the incentive to market to high-risk groups or to oversell. However, merit increases may be awarded. The director of marketing commented that they do not like to appear "too salesy." There are no quotas as such, although each representative develops performance targets. For example, enrolling between 15 and 20 new groups a year is considered to be good performance.

Consumer Relations

Lifeguard's consumer and professional relations department (CPRD) handles inquiries from subscribers, employers, physicians, and occasionally, hospitals. However, the principal role of the department is to address member questions and complaints, since the majority of provider issues surface through other channels, such as CHAP.

The organizational locus of the department is unusual. It is under the executive staff member whose primary role is to negotiate with hospitals, implement the CHAP hospital review program, and monitor all institutional care. Consumer relations or member services functions are typically independent or under the marketing department.

Organization and Function

The department sees itself as the hub of a wheel, because it interacts with all other departments. The purpose of CPRD, according to the department supervisor, is to provide correct information to callers while projecting a professional, yet warm and positive, attitude.

The equivalent of 8.5 full-time employees works at CPRD and handles 1,600 to 1,700 calls per week. The average call lasts 8 to 10 minutes. The goal is to provide good service, which takes time; productivity is not stressed. Consumer representatives are encouraged to give their names and to invite callers to telephone back if they encounter further difficulty.

New members are not contacted routinely; CPRD believes this would not be worthwhile, since only a fraction of new members needs help understanding the Lifeguard system. Feedback to other departments is informal rather than structured. Although the number of calls is recorded, a tally of the nature of each call or the problems reported is no longer maintained.

Problems

Job burnout and high turnover have been a problem. The job of consumer representative is stressful because it entails dealing with unhappy members, often in situations where payment for services has been denied. Two steps have been taken to alleviate this problem. First, each representative has one hour per day off the telephone to research questions raised by enrollees, make follow-up calls, and complete paperwork. Second, an early morning staff meeting is held once or twice a month, on employee time, to discuss problems, try to achieve consistency, and review the plan's contractual obligations.

Another problem is communicating with non-English-speaking or less educated members who do not understand the plan's literature. The CPRD supervisor is the only person in the department who speaks Spanish. As an additional step, the department's staff believes that Lifeguard's literature should be bilingual.

New Directions

Lifeguard is investigating the possibility of creating a consumer response center with a computerized telephone-answering system. The system would work as follows:

— A member would call in during regular hours, describe a problem requiring research to a representative, and be given a case number.

— The member would then call back later (with 24-hour access), punch in the case number using a push-button telephone, and get a recorded answer.

The goal of such a system is to improve efficiency by handling many routine calls with stock answers and to eliminate the stress on representatives by reducing their burden. Implementing the response center concept, however, would also reduce the amount of personal attention that callers now receive.

Organizational Philosophy and Business Operations

In any large-scale enterprise, success depends on good policymaking and management at all levels, from strategic planning to the day-to-day operations associated with paying claims, answering inquiries from members and providers, and so forth. In this section, we discuss selected aspects of Lifeguard's organizational philosophy and approach to business operations, specifically the organizational culture, the role of the board, and financial performance and rate setting.

Organizational Culture

Lifeguard is characterized by at least three distinctive features: strong ties to physicians, a belief in locally managed fee-for-service medicine, and a businesslike yet personal approach to operations.

Strong Ties to Physicians. Physicians are one of Lifeguard's major constituents, due in large part to the philosophy of the plan's founders and to its origins as a foundation for medical care. These foundations typically share three basic beliefs, and the influence of each is evident at Lifeguard:

— Physicians must retain responsibility and leadership in the design, administration, and delivery of medical services.

— Medical care must be provided at a just and equitable cost to both patient and physician.

— Peer review must be encouraged as an efficient mechanism for controlling the rise of medical costs.

The ties to organized medicine are also strong. For example, Lifeguard president Robert Burnett is a former president of the Santa Clara County Medical Society and is an active member of the American Medical Association, which recently elected him to its council on medical services. Six of the seven physician members of the Lifeguard board have served as president of the Santa Clara County Foundation for Medical Care.

Locally Managed, Fee-for-Service System. Underlying the operations of Lifeguard is the philosophy that the fee-for-service system merits preservation and, furthermore, that having the bulk of medical care in the United States delivered through a dozen or so large national entities, whether proprietary or nonprofit, is not in the best interest of patients. At the same time, Lifeguard itself is expanding into other communities and believes that such expansion is important for the plan's financial stability.

Businesslike yet Personal Approach. While the plan functions in a businesslike atmosphere, a personal touch pervades it. This to some extent reflects Dorothy Emerson's personality and philosophy. On the one hand, she says that "culture does not matter any more—dollars do," but on the other hand, she knows many Lifeguard physicians well from her early years in the business, and employees display strong personal loyalty to her.

The businesslike aspects of Lifeguard have already been described—speedy claims payment, no-nonsense utilization review, and so forth. The personal aspects are more intangible, but some examples can be cited. Management welcomes employee ideas for improvements and listens to complaints; there is an informal policy that "no question is a stupid question"; and all staff are encouraged to understand the big picture whenever possible. Close relations with physicians is another example, although, predictably, growth is having an adverse effect on these. In particular, physicians no longer find it as easy to call up Burnett or Emerson and ask for an explanation or a change in policy. As Emerson said, "We have about 2,000 doctors now, and they no longer feel as though Lifeguard is *their* plan."

The CHAP nurses take steps to maintain rapport with participating hospital utilization review nurses, and CPRD telephone representatives are urged to give their names to callers and provide as much personal service as possible. Finally, Lifeguard's staff is still small enough (about 70 people) to preserve the feeling of individual involvement. An outside board member reported that Emerson has generated strong loyalties among staff members, as evidenced by low turnover.

Role of the Board

Lifeguard has a self-perpetuating 14-person board. New bylaws require that one-third of the board members be subscribers and two-thirds providers (physicians and hospital representatives). The board typically meets bimonthly for three to six hours; a five-member executive committee meets more frequently. The plan recently began to pay board members for their service.

The role of the board is to set broad policy, for example to review expansion plans and decide on coverage. The board recently discussed coverage of amniocentesis and organ transplants. Before each meeting, the board routinely receives membership and utilization statistics as well as income statements and balance sheets. One highly controversial issue that received considerable attention last year was whether the plan should convert to for-profit status. Doing so would have made raising capital easier and would have facilitated the introduction of profit-related incentives for senior staff members, consistent with steps taken by many other HMOs. Ultimately, the board decided to remain nonprofit, largely because of opposition from physicians, who felt that converting would be antithetical to the plan's mission. Also, the state of California would have required an initial capitalization from retained earnings in excess of $7 million. An issue currently being addressed is whether to be licensed as an insurer rather than as an HMO. The major advantage of the change is that the plan would not need state approval every time it sought to expand its service area.

Two employers serve on the board and help bring to it the perspective of employers and employees. One such board member indicated continuing employee discontent with mental health and substance abuse services, although he also reported receiving far fewer employee complaints about Lifeguard and other local HMOs than he does for the company's self-insured indemnity plan. The employers also bring a business and financial perspective and have been instrumental in addressing issues relating to financial planning, marketing, and compensation structures.

Financial Performance and Rate Setting

The overall financial philosophy of the plan has been a conservative one. This is reflected in rate setting. It is also reflected in the underwriting practices of the plan, which include not covering large categories of employers such as retail outlets and hospitals. Finally, the investment policy for reserves is a conservative one; cash is invested mostly in short-term bank certificates of deposit.

The plan uses strict community rating, except that it charges individual enrollees (who convert from group coverage) roughly 15 percent more than group enrollees because of higher administrative costs. In some cases, premiums are adjusted to reflect the average family size of a group. In the early days of the plan, rate setting was based largely on actuarial studies. More recently, it has been based on projections from past experience combined with an assessment of what the market will bear.

Premiums have traditionally been set high enough to generate strong reserves, with the surplus reaching a record high of $3.2 million on a revenue base of $32.8 million in 1984 (see table 18.4). Historically, Lifeguard's premiums have been higher than Kaiser's. In the early years, Lifeguard's premiums increased by more than 10 percent annually, but for the last 18 months increases have been held to less than 5 percent. This reflects the need to stay competitive in an increasingly crowded market and the desire not to generate excessive surpluses. Currently, Life-

Table 18.4

Summary of Lifeguard's Revenues and Expenses, 1981–1984

	Fiscal Year*			
	1981 ($1,000s)	1982 ($1,000s)	1983 ($1,000s)	1984 ($1,000s)
Revenues				
Premiums	6,409	12,765	20,953	31,718
Provider membership fees	117	114	48	55
Interest income	318	600	623	1,025
Total	6,844	13,479	21,624	32,798
Expenses				
Health care services	5,697	10,818	17,582	26,747
Other (mostly administrative)	1,048	1,466	1,817	2,885
Total	6,745	12,284	19,399	29,632
Surplus	99	1,195	2,225	3,166

Source: Audited financial statements for the various years.

* The fiscal year ends June 30.

guard's premiums relative to Kaiser's, for a three-way rate structure, are a follows:

Plan	One Person	Two Persons	Three Persons
Lifeguard	$75.50	$151.00	$207.25
Kaiser	$69.01	$137.02	$197.87

The plan does reinsure for very large expenses. Currently, the reinsurance company pays 90 percent of expenses over $85,000 per enrollee per year.

19

Success Factors

While many aspects of Lifeguard's operations have clearly contributed to its success, four are especially striking: early entry into the market with a broad physician panel, outstanding utilization review, good physician relations, and careful, hands-on management.

Early Entry into the Market

Lifeguard was the first broad-based IPA to enter the Santa Clara Valley market. It offers members a cross-section of community physicians, including solo practitioners, physicians in small groups, and a few large and prominent multispecialty groups. Although Kaiser predated Lifeguard by many years, Lifeguard's open-panel model was the first to allow people to receive comprehensive prepaid health benefits from participating private practice physicians. Lifeguard thus occupies a different niche from group- or staff-model HMOs. Also, since employers under Title XIII of the Public Health Service Act can be mandated to offer one IPA or network HMO as well as one group or staff HMO, Lifeguard had the advantage of gaining access to many employer groups that were already familiar with the HMO concept because of the longstanding presence of Kaiser.

Utilization Review

Particularly because physicians are not at risk as individuals, cost management through utilization review has been critical. There are three components to utilization review at Lifeguard: hospital preadmission and concurrent review, a computerized review of claims before payment, and retrospective review of utilization profiles. Together, these programs represent a comprehensive, state-of-the-art system for monitoring and controlling health care utilization. Inpatient ancillary services are the only significant aspect of utilization not addressed by Lifeguard's system; however, tracking these services for hospitals on a per diem basis is less important, because they are usually included in the per diem rate. Since the details of the system have been covered earlier, suffice it to say that few HMOs have as much knowledge of service utilization or the ability to act on such knowledge in a timely fashion.

An important feature is that physicians are automatically provided with feedback as soon as the plan's review system identifies possible overutilization, even if no claims are denied. Thus, physicians always know where they stand and when they should be prepared to justify a pattern of utilization that appears to be beyond normal bounds.

Good Relations with Physicians

Lifeguard recognizes that, in some sense, physicians are its product. The plan therefore places high priority on physician satisfaction. Lifeguard physicians are the first line of contact with members, and disgruntled physicians will, in the opinion of Dorothy Emerson, result in dissatisfied members.

It is remarkable that Lifeguard is able to maintain the high degree of control over utilization described above without incurring resentment among physicians. While confrontations can and do occur from time to time, they are minimized by adherence to two cardinal rules: pay promptly, and pay reasonable fees.

Careful Management

Finally, Lifeguard executives pay close personal attention to daily business. Top managers are involved in operations, accessible, and committed. Lifeguard is thus able to provide a style of health care delivery that is highly acceptable to consumers and fee-for-service providers without breaking the budget.

Part V

Harvard Community Health Plan

20

Introduction

Harvard Community Health Plan (HCHP) is a federally qualified, nonprofit, staff-model HMO with headquarters in Boston, Massachusetts. The plan began operations in October 1969 and now serves over 200,000 members from 115 cities and towns in the Boston area. It operates eight health centers and its own 69-bed hospital. It recently entered into a contractual relationship with Brigham and Women's Hospital, one of the teaching hospitals of the Harvard Medical School, under which the hospital will commit a substantial number of beds to HCHP at a discounted daily rate.

One of the earliest and largest HMOs in New England, HCHP has experienced remarkably consistent annual growth (see table 20.1). Most of the enrollees are members of about 2,200 employer groups served by HCHP; 1,400 of these groups have 25 or more HCHP members. Within the last two years, HCHP has begun to cultivate small employer groups, too. It has added a SeniorCare program for Medicare beneficiaries which now accounts for 2,400 members.

Financial performance has been excellent since 1980, except in 1981, when a hospital cost overrun caused a net loss for the year (see table 20.2).

Table 20.1

HCHP Membership

Fiscal Year	Members
1970	5,000
1972	28,900
1974	40,100
1976	60,000
1978	78,700
1980	98,300
1982	126,600
1984	178,200
1985	204,700

Table 20.2

Income Statement for HCHP, 1980–1984

	Fiscal Year*				
	1980 ($1,000s)	1981 ($1,000s)	1982 ($1,000s)	1983 ($1,000s)	1984 ($1,000s)
Revenues					
Member premiums	44,487	57,345	69,931	99,540	128,612
Other	4,125	5,822	6,097	6,683	10,358
Total	48,612	63,167	76,028	106,223	138,970
Expenses					
Salaries and wages	16,188	21,547	26,124	32,330	41,442
Fringe benefits	2,618	3,439	4,635	6,148	8,620
Research grants	209	342	182	310	536
Interest	799	1,407	1,554	1,935	2,018
Depreciation	1,363	1,751	1,711	2,868	3,602
Hospital services	13,518	21,042	23,136	29,466	38,002
Other	11,088	14,924	15,525	26,462	36,775
Total	45,783	64,452	72,867	99,519	130,995
Surplus (deficit)	2,829	(1,285)†	3,161†	6,704	7,975

* The fiscal year ends September 30.
† Fiscal year 1982 reflects an $825,000 reinsurance recovery relating to the 1981 hospital cost overrun.

21

The Market

The economic and demographic characteristics of HCHP's service area are mixed with respect to the potential for HMO development. Although the population is affluent and well educated, it is growing more slowly than in other parts of the United States (except in suburban areas) and has a higher age distribution. Medical cost, utilization, and supply factors are favorable for HMO development; utilization rates and expenses per capita are high, the bed supply is more than adequate, and there is an excess supply of physicians. The health insurance market has not been competitive in the past but is increasingly becoming so.

Data are presented by county, when available, to mirror the HCHP service area precisely; otherwise, metropolitan statistical area data for greater Boston are substituted.

Economic and Demographic Characteristics

The HCHP service area is composed of five counties encircling Boston, falling largely within the Route 495 interstate highway. It thus encompasses all of Boston, Cambridge, the Route 128 engineering and computer firms, and many of the outlying small towns and suburban areas.

The five-county area has almost 3.7 million people (see table 21.1). In the aggregate, the service area is growing less rapidly than the U.S. average of 11.4 percent. The three largest counties (Middlesex, Suffolk, and Essex) all declined in size between 1970 and 1980. The most suburban county (Plymouth) grew by nearly 22 percent.

Table 21.1

Population and Socioeconomic Characteristics of the HCHP Service Area

County	1980 Population	Change Since 1970 (%)	Over Age 65, 1983 (%)	Median Family Income, 1979 ($)	Below Poverty Level, 1979 (%)	Unemployment Rate, April 1985 (%)	High School Graduates, 1983 (%)
Essex	633,632	− .7	13.3	21,660	9.1	3.7	73.0
Middlesex	1,367,034	− 2.2	11.6	24,039	7.0	2.7	77.4
Norfolk	606,587	.3	12.7	25,434	5.5	2.9	82.0
Plymouth	405,437	21.6	10.5	21,317	8.0	4.4	77.1
Suffolk	650,142	−11.6	13.0	16,443	19.1	4.3	67.8
Total	3,662,832						
U.S. Average		11.4	11.7	16,841	12.4	7.1	66.5

Source: U.S. Department of Commerce, Bureau of the Census, *County and City Data Book—1983* (Washington, D.C.: Government Printing Office, 1983); U.S. Department of Labor, Bureau of Labor Statistics, personal communication.

The service area population is older than the national average of 11.7 percent over age 65. Three of the five counties are considerably above the U.S. average; Essex has the oldest population with 13.3 percent over 65. Only one county, Plymouth, is significantly below the U.S. average, with 10.5 percent of its population over age 65.

The area is an affluent one, with low overall poverty and unemployment rates. Median incomes in 1979 ranged from $16,443 in Suffolk county (Boston) to $25,434 in Norfolk County, 51 percent above the U.S. median of $16,841. The poverty rate in 1979 was considerably below the national average of 12.4 percent in all counties except Suffolk, where at 19.1 percent it is much higher. Unemployment rates are very low, ranging from 2.7 percent to 4.4 percent in April 1985, compared to the U.S. average of 7.1 percent in the same month. Finally, the population is well educated—all counties are above the U.S. norm for the percentage completing secondary school.

Medical Utilization, Cost, and Supply Factors

The Boston medical market is rather unrestrained, with utilization rates and per capita medical expenses above average for all U.S. metropolitan areas. Boston's status as a major teaching and tertiary referral center clearly contributes to higher costs and utilization and has also drawn a large number of physicians to the area.

Utilization data for the Boston MSA compared to the U.S. average for metropolitan areas show that Boston was above the norm on every measure in 1983 (see table 21.2):

— Inpatient days per thousand persons in Boston were 20 percent higher than the U.S. metropolitan average.

— Admissions were 4 percent higher.

— Average length of stay was 14 percent higher.

— The occupancy rate was 12 percent higher.

Reflecting the pattern of high utilization and the disproportionately high number of teaching hospitals, physician and hospital bed supply are also high. The greater Boston area has 70 percent more physicians than the national average (see table 21.3). Physician supply ranges greatly, from 1.2 M.D.'s per thousand persons in rural Plymouth County to 7.6 in Suffolk, where three

Table 21.2

Medical Utilization, Cost, and Supply Factors in the Boston Standard Metropolitan Statistical Area, 1983

Factor	Boston MSA*	Average for MSAs
Inpatient days per 1,000 persons	1,453	1,206
Admissions per 1,000 persons	166	159
Hospital beds per 1,000 persons	4.8	4.5
Average length of stay (days)	8.7	7.6
Occupancy rate (%)	82.6	74
Hospital expenses per capita ($)	884	560

Source: American Hospital Association, *Hospital Statistics* (Chicago: AHA, 1984); U.S. Department of Commerce, Bureau of the Census, *Statistical Abstract of the United States—1985* (Washington, D.C.: Government Printing Office, 1984).

* The population of the Boston MSA totals 2,804,000; this includes Suffolk county and parts of Bristol, Essex, Middlesex, Norfolk, Plymouth, and Worcester counties.

Table 21.3

Supply of M.D.'s in HCHP's Service Area, 1983

County	M.D.'s	Population	M.D.'s per 1,000 Persons
Essex	1,108	641,000	1.7
Middlesex	4,487	1,366,000	3.3
Norfolk	2,366	604,000	3.9
Plymouth	515	418,000	1.2
Suffolk	4,880	644,000	7.6
Total	13,356	3,673,000	3.6
United States	501,958	233,981,000	2.1

Sources: American Medical Association, personal communication; U.S. Department of Commerce, Bureau of the Census, *Statistical Abstract of the United States—1985* (Washington, D.C.: Government Printing Office, 1984).

medical schools are based (Harvard, Tufts, and Boston University).[1] The supply of hospital beds per thousand persons is only slightly above the metropolitan area norm—4.8 in the Boston MSA compared to 4.5 in all MSAs.

Given the above data, it is not surprising that hospital expenses per capita are high in the Boston MSA. (Data for the five counties comprising HCHP's service area are not available.) Per capita expenses in 1983 were 58 percent higher than the U.S. MSA average (see table 21.2).

The Health Insurance Market

The health insurance market in Boston traditionally was not highly competitive, and HCHP operated for several years under an indemnity plan price umbrella. In the last few years, competition among HMOs has accelerated as more plans have followed HCHP into the market. Blue Cross–Blue Shield (BC-BS) insures about 65 percent of the greater Boston market, while other commercial insurance companies serve another 20 percent. Twelve HMOs together claim about 15 percent of the market.

Of the 11 other HMOs in the greater Boston area, two are available only to employees and dependents of the sponsoring universities (MIT Health Plan and Harvard University Group Health Plan). Major competitors of HCHP include Bay State Health Care, Multigroup Health Plan, Tufts Associated Health Plan, and three plans affiliated with BC-BS—Healthway Medical Plan, Lahey Clinic Health Plan, and Medical East Community Health Plan (see table 21.4). Other major HMOs in New England that compete regionally include another BC-BS affiliate, Fallon Community Health Plan in Worcester, Massachusetts; Rhode Island Group Health Association in Providence; and Community Health Care Plan in New Haven, Connecticut.

The Boston HMO market is a relatively young one. Although the largest of its local competitors is only half the size of HCHP, many of the newcomers are open-panel plans, which can expand quickly, and they are targeting the lower cost, faster growing suburban areas. Some indications of the rapid changes taking place are the following:

— In the last five years, seven new HMOs started up in Boston.

— In three and one-half years, Multigroup Health Plan, based in Wellesley, grew from 2,600 to 48,600 members.

— Massachusetts Blue Cross–Blue Shield has one of the best and most competitive HMO development programs in the country and currently is affiliated with or sponsoring four HMOs in HCHP's service area.

Table 21.4

HCHP's Service Area in HMOs

Plan	Year Formed	Model	Members	
			June 1981	December 1984
Harvard Community Health Plan Boston	1969	Staff	107,724	184,031
Bay State Health Care Cambridge	1979	IPA	18,570	97,500
Multigroup Health Plan Wellesley	1980	Network	2,636	48,588
Tufts Associated Health Plan Waltham	1981	IPA	—	34,200
Healthway Medical Plan* Brockton	1979	Group	6,381	32,600
Lahey Clinic–BCBS Health Plan* Burlington	1980	Group	4,981	24,164
Family Health Plan of Massachusetts Framingham	1982	IPA	—	19,033

Table 21.4—continued

HMOs in HCHP's Service Area

Plan	Year Formed	Model	Members	
			June 1981	December 1984
Medical East Community Health Plan* Chicopee	1982	Staff	—	16,161
MIT Health Plan Cambridge	1973	Staff	7,450	8,532
West Suburban Health Care Plan* Waltham	1980	IPA	1,347	7,500
Harvard University Group Health Plan Cambridge	1972	Staff	5,112	6,293
Boston Health Plan* Boston	1981	Network	—	6,252
Total			154,201	484,854

Source: Modified from InterStudy, *National HMO Census, 1981* (Excelsior, Minn.: InterStudy, 1981) and *National HMO Census, 1984* (Excelsior, Minn.: InterStudy, 1985).

* Affiliated with or sponsored by Blue Cross–Blue Shield Massachusetts.

— No commercially marketed HMO other than HCHP is
more than six years old.

HCHP has captured 7 to 8 percent of the market within its
service area. Despite one senior executive's remark that "We are
not the IBM of HMOs," HCHP is preeminent in Boston, and
studies show its name recognition with consumers is exception-
ally high, on the order of 85 percent. While PPOs and proprietary
hospital chains offering health insurance products are not a threat
in the Boston area so far, HCHP does have competitive concerns.
The plan notes that as BC-BS loses market share, it is becoming
more aggressive in developing new products; HCHP believes BC-
BS has deep pockets, which enhances its ability to compete. The
plan was also concerned that its higher rates were impeding enrollment in outlying areas, where suburban-based HMOs using
less expensive community hospitals can charge lower rates. To alleviate this problem, the plan recently applied for and received
approval from the Office of HMOs to create a subregional component with a different rate structure on the outer fringe of the
plan's current service area. Finally, HCHP believes that it needs
to develop a strategy to retain national account business in the
face of multistate HMO competitors. The plan's current strategy is
to increase its capacity to serve regional firms in New England.

Note

1. Data on physician supply in the United States are for the entire country; metropolitan areas would be expected to have a denser physician
population. Suffolk County, however, has more physicians per thousand persons than most other urban centers, such as San Francisco
County (6.8) or Philadelphia County (3.8).

22

Overview

$\mathbf{A}$ nonprofit health plan founded in 1969 and federally qualified in 1977, HCHP is the oldest and largest HMO in New England. It was initiated by Harvard Medical School but has always been a separate, independent corporation. It continues to be affiliated with Harvard Medical School: it admits members to Harvard teaching hospitals, many of its physicians hold teaching appointments at the medical school, and a commitment has been made to share resources related to education and medical care between the two institutions.

As the first HMO developed by an academic medical center, HCHP was—and continues to be—experimental. Robert H. Ebert, then dean of Harvard Medical School and now chairman of HCHP's board of overseers, believed prepaid group practice could contribute to the mission of a medical school in the following ways:[1]

— Provide a core population for teaching and research

— Increase access to care for the underserved

— Control costs, thereby benefiting society economically

— Test innovative health service programs

Planning and early implementation were handled by members of the dean's staff. Physician services and inpatient care were negotiated with the major Harvard teaching hospitals. Marketing was conducted by Blue Cross and other insurers, without great success. The plan's first health center opened in 1969 with only 88 members (see table 22.1), yet enough staff for 10,000 enrollees had been hired.

Initial funding was in the form of grants and loans from various sources, including the federal government, the Ford Foundation, the Commonwealth Fund, and the Harvard Corporation. The plan lost almost $2.9 million in its first three years and operated in the black for the first time in December 1972, with over 30,000 members.

In the early 1970s, HCHP was still a "patchwork system of contracts," according to one executive. The plan depended heavily on the Harvard teaching hospitals for physicians and on Blue Cross and commercial carriers for marketing and insurance functions. Still, its leaders had a strong desire to innovate, even at this stage, and HCHP developed a broad benefits package, began an automated medical records system, and experimented with an expanded role for nurses.

Enrolling new members was a major priority; therefore, the plan began to rely less on third-party payers to sell HCHP to employers and more on its own staff. In about 1972, the first physicians were brought onto HCHP's payroll. Increased marketing efforts began to pay off, and in 1973 HCHP opened a new health center in Cambridge. At this point, there was a risk of splitting the organization into two physician groups, but the executive director at the time held firmly to the belief that the Cambridge Center must remain part of the system. Growth continued over the next few years, and in 1975–76 the plan broke off with Blue Cross and the commercial carriers and took control of marketing and enrollment.

Another turning point came in 1978–79, when HCHP took over the operations of the Parker Hill Medical Center, now HCHP Hospital. The hospital gives the plan access to beds for secondary care, and, in return, the plan has significantly helped the hospital budget. The Wellesley Center opened in 1980, giving HCHP three delivery sites, and total enrollment surpassed 100,000.

Then, in 1981, the plan suffered a setback: it experienced both a significant increase in hospital days per thousand persons and a jump in the average inpatient cost per day, resulting in a loss of $1,285,000. The shortfall was not observed until 1982, due to an inadequate approach to calculating claims incurred but not received (IBNRs). As a result, HCHP improved its method of estimating IBNRs and tightened concurrent review in the hospital. Nearly two-thirds of the loss was later recouped in reinsurance payments.

In retrospect, one sees that this difficult period helped prepare HCHP for the increasingly competitive environment in which it would be operating after 1981. Over the last few years, the plan has felt greater pressure to examine its wage policies, staffing, and hospital contracting arrangements in order to keep its cost structure, and therefore premiums, competitive. As it opened more suburban health centers, the plan began using community hospitals in addition to Harvard teaching institutions, both for greater cost control and for patient convenience. HCHP has continued to thrive and add new centers, expanding to Medford and Braintree in 1982 and opening centers in Peabody and downtown Boston in 1984.

The plan continues to grow and change. In 1984 it formed Managed Care, a for-profit affiliate, to develop, own, and manage open-panel HMOs and other alternative delivery systems outside HCHP's service area. Managed Care took four managers from HCHP, and HCHP nominates candidates for four of seven seats on its board. The president of HCHP currently serves as chairman. In 1985, after more than two years of development and preparation, HCHP signed a Medicare risk contract with the Health Care Financing Administration and began enrolling beneficiaries in SeniorCare. HCHP recently announced it has reached an agreement in principle with Brigham and Women's Hospital, a major Harvard teaching center, to rely on that hospital for a significant portion of inpatient days.

Values

There is a distinct HCHP culture, and it is manifested in shared values. Plan executives and staff exhibit a strong desire to be the best and to make a difference. They believe that HCHP *does* excel and take tangible pride in its accomplishments. The plan's first heart transplant recipient, Knut Seeber, became a symbol of the plan's achievements to many staff members and was featured in the 1984 annual report.

One expression of the plan's values—and one frequently referred to—is the HCHP diamond. Its four points are service, quality, cost containment, and staff development. The goal is to balance these four objectives. A staff recognition program makes HCHP diamond awards to selected employees each year.

The plan has a strategic planning process, described in greater detail later in this chapter, in which it regularly examines

Table 22.1

Significant Events in the Development of HCHP

Year	Event
1969	HCHP opens Kenmore Center with 88 members.
1970	Medicaid contract signed with Massachusetts Department of Public Welfare; satellite center at Mission Hill opens to serve this population, with subsequent support from the U.S. Public Health Service.
1971	Law passed to allow state and local public employees to join HCHP.
1972	In December, HCHP operates in the black for the first time; automated medical records system operational; dental program started.
1973	Temporary Cambridge Center opens.
1974	Kenmore Center membership exceeds capacity; controls instituted to limited enrollment.
1975	Permanent Cambridge Center opens; HCHP Medicare supplement program begins.
1976	Arrangement with Blue Cross for marketing and enrollment is severed; HCHP allocates 1.25% of premiums to research, education, and community service; new prepaid drug benefit offered; optical service begins; letter of understanding between HCHP and Harvard Medical School provides for cooperation in programs of mutual interest.
1977	HCHP becomes federally qualified.
1978	Agreement with Parker Hill Medical Center gives HCHP operating control and guaranteed access to beds.
1979	Parker Hill generates a surplus and saves HCHP over $200,000 in hospital costs.

Table 22.1—continued

Significant Events in the Development of HCHP

Year	Event
1980	HCHP Foundation formed to support activities in teaching, research, and community service; Wellesley Center opens; Office of HMOs approves a $1.68 million grant to equip the Wellesley and Medford centers; enrollment exceeds 100,000.
1981	Mission Hill (Medicaid) members transferred to Kenmore Center due to loss of federal funding; HCHP runs a year-end deficit of $1,285,000.
1982	Parker Hill renamed the HCHP Hospital; Medford and Braintree Centers open.
1983	HCHP's research department merges with Harvard School of Public Health's Center for the Analysis of Health Practices to form the Institute for Health Research; HCHP announces it will cover heart and liver transplants; first HCHP conference for nurse practitioners is held; psychiatric day treatment program started.
1984	Peabody and Boston centers open; first public debt offering raises $49 million for health center construction and renovation; primary nursing initiated at HCHP Hospital; Managed Care formed; physician recruitment office opens.
1985	SeniorCare program (Medicare risk contract) enrolls first beneficiaries; new agreement with Brigham and Women's Hospital signed.

issues in light of plan values. One such issue is growth. Growth is a recurring subject, and one that engenders strong feelings on every side. When HCHP asks itself why it should grow, purely financial goals are dismissed early on. Decisions to grow have been based on a desire to serve more people ("to provide our style of care in new communities," according to one executive) and to protect market share. This blending of both service and business objectives is characteristic of HCHP.

The ability to combine the plan's academic roots and its teaching, research, and community service objectives with sound business practice is a tribute to HCHP's basic values. The plan has adapted over time, while preserving the HCHP diamond. The remaining sections of this chapter cover the specifics of plan operations.

Benefits and Coverage

About 88 percent of HCHP's members are from about 2,200 employer groups. The rest of the membership is comprised of non-group enrollees and Medicare and Medicaid beneficiaries. HCHP offers one basic benefit package to all employer groups; the variations in coverage for other components of HCHP's membership are not discussed here. Benefits are comprehensive; routine care, including preventive services, is virtually unlimited, and cost sharing is minimal. All nonemergency care must be provided or authorized by an HCHP clinician in order to be covered.

Outpatient benefits include diagnostic and treatment services, adult and pediatric health examinations, eye and hearing examinations, immunizations and injections, medical social services, family planning, maternal care, up to 20 mental health visits per year, alcohol and drug detoxification, and preventive dental care (for children under age 12 only). Covered inpatient services include unlimited acute-care days, all physician and ancillary services, blood transfusion services (excluding blood and blood products), and special-duty nursing when ordered by an HCHP clinician. In addition, the plan covers essential ambulance service and both in-area and out-of-area emergency care. Other special services covered include:

— Hemodialysis, whether inpatient, outpatient, or at home
— Human organ transplant (heart, liver, cornea, kidney, and heart-lung)

— Noncustodial extended care up to 100 days, including prescribed drugs and ancillary services

— Home health care when essential to treatment and obtained from an HCHP-designated provider (medical services only)

— Short-term physical therapy and rehabilitation services, whether inpatient, outpatient, or at home

— Inpatient mental health services up to 60 days per year

— Certain durable medical equipment and corrective appliances, in accordance with various specifications and restrictions

The standard copayment for outpatient services is $3. This copayment is charged for outpatient, including mental health, visits and prescriptions ($3 for a 30-day supply). No copayment is required for home health or physical therapy services or for any aspect of inpatient care. The copayment for scheduled after-hours visits is $5; that for the annual preventive dental visit under age 12, $8. If HCHP chooses to provide hemodialysis services in a member's home, the plan will cover the costs of installing necessary equipment, up to $300. Fees are charged for some health education programs.

The principal exclusions are eyeglasses, contact lenses, and hearing aids; biofeedback, acupuncture, and chiropractic services; transsexual surgery; reversal of voluntary sterilization; any services not necessary for the protection of a member's health; and experimental procedures, unless approved by HCHP's board of directors.

The major supplemental benefit is outpatient prescription drugs, and 75 percent of employers opt for it. The plan believes that variable benefit packages are increasingly popular, and, to remain competitive, it is likely to develop a low option and more variations in the existing package of services.

For its decisions about offering services not mandated by federal or state law, HCHP's benefits and contracts committee has developed evaluation criteria. These are

— Member and staff expectations

— Risk of adverse selection

— Cost-effectiveness

— "Value" of the service

The committee also considers any benefit issue in light of three organizational values: equity, comprehensive coverage, and affordability.

Two coverage decisions illustrate the application of these principles.[2] In 1983, HCHP decided to cover heart and liver transplants. To summarize the evaluation process, heart and liver transplants are important services that members and staff felt should be covered; the risk of adverse selection exists but is tempered by the fact that patients cannot delay the service while changing insurance; the cost is about $100,000, with a one-year survival rate of 70 to 80 percent; and the services have great value since they are usually a last resort. The case of in vitro fertilization provides a counterpoint: staff would like to cover the procedure, but, although individual members have sought coverage, there is little demand from the membership as a whole; the risk of adverse selection is great; the cost per attempt is $5,000, and only about 10 percent of attempts are successful; and the value of the service is great, but life-enhancing rather than life-prolonging.

Although the decision to exclude in vitro fertilization was difficult, the committee felt HCHP's organizational values added further justification. The cost to the total membership of covering in vitro fertilization was expected to be great (greater than the cost of covering heart and liver transplants because of the higher incidence of in vitro fertilization procedures), while the cost to the individual is more attainable than the cost of transplants. These factors, combined with the risk of adverse selection, high rate of failure, and small impact on health, helped confirm the decision. The plan expects to reexamine the issue again, however, as success rates and costs change.

Delivery of Services

Three new health centers are planned for 1986–88. The new centers will be smaller (capacity of 12–30,000 members) and located in more suburban areas than the eight existing centers (see table 22.2). All primary care physicians and many specialists are on staff, based in the health centers. Laboratory, X-ray, pharmacy, and optical (Kenmore only) services are available on-site. HCHP Hospital, not far from the Kenmore Center, completes the internal network. An urgent and after-hours visit unit is located at HCHP Hospital.[3] In addition to HCHP's own hospital, the plan is affiliated with 14 other hospitals in the Boston area.

Table 22.2

Current and Planned HCHP Health Centers,
Membership, and Capacity

Health Center (Year Opened)	Capacity	Members April 30, 1985
Current		
Kenmore (1969)	58,000	53,905
Cambridge (1973)	40,000	40,492
Wellesley (1980)	40,000	29,938
Medford (1982)	37,500	25,929
Braintree (1982)	30,000	19,598
Peabody (1984)	30,000	7,785
Boston (1984)	30,000	15,680
Southborough (1985)	12,500	—
Subtotal	278,000	193,327
Planned		
West Roxbury (4/86)	25,000	
Watertown (7/87–7/88)	22,000	
Additional West Centers (7/87–7/88)	12,500	
Subtotal	62,500	
Total	340,500	193,327

Members of HCHP are required to sign up with a particular health center. To help them decide which one, they receive information on the principal hospital affiliations of each center, as well as its affiliations for emergency referral and selected specialty services. Next, members are given a brochure to help them choose a primary care physician at that center. The brochure lists each primary care physician (internal medicine, pediatrics, or obstetrics/gynecology) and the nurse practitioner with whom he or she practices. In addition, a book listing every physician on staff at HCHP, by health center, is available; it provides the specialty, medical school attended, year of graduation, and location of internship and residency programs.

Medical Staff

The plan employs 271 full-time physicians. This includes 103 internists, 39 pediatricians, 30 psychiatrists, 29 obstetricians, 15 surgeons, 10 orthopedists, 10 ophthalmologists, and 35 other subspecialists. The plan also employs 19 psychologists with Ph.D.'s and a number of part-time physicians who practice in the after-hours clinic. Physician turnover has been a stable 4 percent over the last three years.

In addition, HCHP has 185 midlevel providers, primarily nurse practitioners and physician assistants, but some mental health counselors as well.

The special relationship HCHP maintains with its staff physicians is an unmistakable outgrowth of the plan's medical school roots.

Physicians' Role

The plan may be unique among HMOs in its strong commitment to using physicians in key management positions.

One mark of this commitment is the organizational stature accorded the medical director. The entire HCHP organization is divided immediately below the president's level into two components, one of which constitutes the health care delivery system. This component is under the unequivocal line authority of the medical director, who also has the title of chief operating officer. (His organizational peer is the executive vice president and chief administrative officer, who directs all "insurance" aspects of the plan and certain planwide administrative functions.) The president and the medical director are the only two HCHP officers who are members of the board of directors.

The significance of the medical director's position is underlined by the fact that he chairs the operations committee, which is composed of essentially all HCHP senior executives. The committee meets every other week and addresses a wide range of operational issues, not solely medical issues. For example, we are told that the operations committee is spending an increasing amount of time discussing marketplace conditions and trends and correspondingly less on how to run various medical specialty practices.

The plan's commitment to the physician-manager concept is most evident, however, in the health centers, the key elements in the delivery system. Each health center is managed by a director, who must be a physician. The health center directors are supported by nonphysician administrators, but the directors' authority over all aspects of health center operations is unequivocal. They function with considerable autonomy.

The four most senior health center directors are designated associate medical directors; three of them have responsibility for overseeing one to three other health centers, and the fourth is responsible for central clinical services (that is, clinical services that are staffed centrally because demand in the centers is not sufficient to justify local staffing).

The medical director's staff also includes a deputy medical director and four physicians in senior staff positions. The only nonphysician in a senior management position under the medical director is the vice president for hospital services, who is a professional hospital administrator.

Thus, management of the HCHP health care delivery system is in the hands of a group of 10 to 15 physicians. Some of these physicians have had management training before being appointed to their positions, including one who earned an M.B.A. Those who have not had such preparation (or who would benefit from more) are sent to executive development programs at leading graduate schools of business—typically Harvard or Stanford. This initial preparation is supplemented by a program of continuing management education.

Top management acknowledges that this is an expensive approach to management staffing but believes that it is justified by the improvements in quality of care, communication between medical and nonmedical staff, competitive position in physician recruitment, and corporate image that result. At the same time, top executives admit that the approach is an experiment, the full results of which will not be known for several years.

The importance of physicians in the HCHP management hierarchy is evidenced also in the existence of the physicians council, which was created in 1982 to respond, in a staff-model context, to the physicians' desire to have an input into corporate policymaking. The physicians council is a committee of the board, and is elected by the physician members of the corporation (staff physicians are eligible to become physician members after five years of service). The council elects two members of the board as well as its own chairperson, who is a member of the policy group.[4] The physicians council has no line authority, but it does advise the board on matters of quality control, reviews hospital programs, proposes the physician compensation plan, participates in the selection of the medical director, approves the appointment of associate medical directors, provides input on benefit changes, and advises on the development of new health centers.

The HCHP medical staff is described as consisting of at least two distinct groups: an old guard—physicians who have been with the plan through most or all of its history—and a new generation of more recently hired physicians. This duality is in part a function of the five-year requirement for becoming a physician member of the corporation and thereby acquiring the right to vote for members of the physicians council. The size of the plan has roughly doubled in the last five years, so there is a considerable number of physicians who have little historical perspective and see themselves as being poorly represented by the physicians council.

The division relates somewhat to concepts of medical care, also. Most of the old guard physicians were and are crusaders for the concept of primary care, in which the primary care physician assumes total responsibility for the medical care of his or her patients. The newer staff physicians are said to be more inclined to assume the specialist role and less willing to take on total responsibility.

Physician Recruitment and Compensation

The plan has high standards for physicians, which can make it difficult to hire them in adequate numbers. The standards are not explicit, but all HCHP physicians must qualify for admitting privileges at a Harvard teaching hospital. Obstetrics-gynecology, orthopedics, and primary care (because of the number of physicians needed) present ongoing recruitment difficulties.

The plan recently created a central physician recruitment office that will contact training programs to publicize available positions. Although HCHP advertises nationally, a high proportion of its recruits was trained at Harvard: about one-third of its physicians went to Harvard Medical School, two-thirds received some or all of their training at Harvard teaching hospitals, and some 85 percent have teaching appointments at Harvard Medical School.

Staff physicians are paid by salary and bonus. Physicians in the same specialty and in the same year of experience are paid equal salaries. Physician salaries are based on the marketplace, which, depending on the specialty, is regional or national. Targets are set for each of the approximately 20 specialties on the staff and are based on physician salary data collected from various sources, including private surveys and professional associations. While subspecialists earn significantly more than primary care physicians, the importance of primary care physicians to the plan is recognized in other ways. For example, HCHP's retirement contributions are capped at the level of primary care physician salaries.

Physicians may be eligible for two types of bonuses. The first is available only to physician members of the corporation, who, as noted above, are physicians with five or more years' service at HCHP. This special status confers such benefits as a low-interest loan program for children's tuition and personal financial planning seminars for physicians and their spouses. Physician members of the corporation also participate in a merit bonus program. This entails an annual performance review, usually at the departmental level, and culminates in bonuses averaging perhaps 5 percent of base salaries. These bonuses are now based on overall health center or departmental performance but will in the future increasingly be based on individual performance.

Second, physicians share in a planwide bonus program. For 11 years, HCHP has been sharing surpluses with all staff through this program. (Two years ago an individual bonus program was started for executives, and they no longer share in the planwide program.) At the end of the year, the board decides what amount will be distributed, based on financial results and other corporate goals. A full share, which is equivalent to approximately 6 percent of eligible staff salaries, is budgeted, but this amount is not paid out if revenues fall short or expenses are too high. Similarly, more than a full share may be paid out in a good year. In 11 years, the distribution has varied from 0 to a 1.75 share. Employees are only entitled to a full share (6 percent of salary) after five years of service; before that, they receive a prorated amount reflecting length of employment.

Bonuses at HCHP have traditionally been related not to individual performance, but to planwide financial success. The plan is moving, however, toward analysis of individual performance—that is, by department and by individual. A proposal to experiment with risk sharing at the new Southborough Center is controversial among physicians. In addition, HCHP recently began to change the bonus program for physician members of the corporation and over three years will phase in a system to reward individual performance in specialties, where appropriate (for example, primary care), and departmental performance, where appropriate (for example, pathology).

The plan as a whole is, in the words of one manager, "ambivalent" about the concept of risk sharing; questions are often asked about what price is paid by setting people in competition with one another while trying to achieve a group goal. Malpractice is another concern that surfaces in discussions about risk sharing.

Utilization Management

Utilization management at HCHP is tied closely to the judgments and needs of clinicians. The plan has not adopted a regulatory approach to utilization control; instead it has developed a sophisticated ambulatory care structure that fosters conservative use of inpatient facilities. In addition, a strong culture contributes to efficient medical practice.

A major objective of the utilization management program, known as the outside health resource utilization program (OHRUP), is to address clinicians' concerns about circumstances in the ambulatory setting that prevent or discourage outpatient treatment. For example, an outpatient oncology unit was created recently to provide chemotherapy services. The unit has comfortable couches, televisions, and other amenities, as well as hospital beds and all the equipment necessary to monitor, hydrate, and nurture patients receiving chemotherapy for a 12-hour period.

The plan does not have a formal authorization process for hospital admissions, but it does require written referral forms for all services not provided within the health centers (including, for example, hospital admissions, consultation with outside specialists, and home care). These referral forms create a record of utilization patterns, but they are not routinely reviewed for clinical appropriateness. In addition, no second opinion is required, although second opinions are available to patients on request. There is a list of procedures that commonly are performed on an outpatient basis, but there is no requirement that they be done so. Preadmission testing is done at the health centers for all routine admissions.

The plan is currently implementing a preferred vendor system. Using the referral forms described above, it has been tracking ten diagnostic tests (including ultrasound, mammograms, evoked potentials, and head and body CAT scans) that are performed outside the health centers to determine utilization rates and cost. Assuming that HCHP decides it is preferable to continue contracting for these services rather than doing them in-house, it will negotiate prices with particular providers. When the program is fully operational, HCHP expects that all referrals will go to preferred vendors unless there are extenuating circumstances. The program will identify preferred vendors for other services as well.

The plan is actively engaged in concurrent review, with five nurse practitioners monitoring HCHP members in the hospital. Reviews often focus on services that lend themselves to alternative levels of care (for example, oncology), certain age groups (for example, the elderly), or selected diagnoses (for example, low back pain). The goal of the concurrent review staff is to make HCHP physicians' lives easier, not to badger them. The nurses seek to avoid inappropriate hospital stays by removing barriers to early discharge and by working with hospital staff to ensure that care is provided at the most efficient level. No length-of-stay norms are used, in part because HCHP's experience is already below most national norms. The plan hopes, however, eventually to develop its own criteria for the appropriateness of hospital services, based on the intensity and severity of illness.

Retrospective analysis of utilization is facilitated by good information systems. The hospital information system creates reports of admissions, discharges, length of stay, and diagnosis by hospital, by primary physician, and by specialty. While aggregated reports of utilization are reviewed by top management, the chiefs of each medical department review more detailed data. Feedback to physicians about utilization patterns thus occurs primarily at the departmental level. On a monthly basis, chiefs receive factual information comparing their departments' performances to the budget with respect to admissions, length of stay, and so on. Although each hospitalization is itemized, individual physicians are not identified. Department chiefs are also supplied with more clinical, subjective information from OHRUP about how patients might have been treated in alternative settings and an explanation of why they were not.

The approach to utilization management is consistent with HCHP's culture and values. The plan is staffed with high-quality physicians who are committed to practicing efficient medicine in an ambulatory care setting; neither regulatory control nor financial incentives has been necessary to deter excess utilization in this environment. HCHP's days of inpatient care per thousand members have been far lower than comparable statistics in the fee-for-service sector since the plan's inception. Hospital utilization has fluctuated from year to year but has remained under 400 days per thousand members (see table 22.3), reaching a low of 343 days per thousand in 1983.

Table 22.3

HCHP Utilization Data

Fiscal Year	Members	Inpatient Days per 1,000 Members*	Health Center Visits per Member
1979	80,500	384	4.2
1980	98,300	367	4.3
1981	110,200	395	4.3
1982	126,600	362	4.3
1983	153,900	343	4.5
1984	178,200	371	4.6
1985	204,700	N.A.	N.A.

* Includes ambulatory surgery, psychiatric day care, and ambulatory abortions.
N.A. indicates data are not available.

Quality Measurement

A vice president for quality measurement has been added to develop measures of quality of care that are analogous to measures of financial performance. To allow an unimpeded flow of information on quality to top management, the vice president reports directly to HCHP's policy group. The staff numbers five and will eventually double. It collects information and works with a quality assurance committee comprised of physicians and nurses.

Quality has been defined broadly under this mandate, with eight dimensions, or indicators, identified thus far. These include two traditional measures, *health outcomes* and *technical process*. A data base is now being installed to provide average birth weight, infant mortality rates, the perinatal complication rate, and a few other outcome-based measures. Reviews to ensure that care conforms to appropriate standards and guidelines, where such standards exist, will monitor technical process. *Access*, including telephone access, appointment and waiting room times, access to emergency care, and access to specialty consultations, is another component of quality that will be regularly assessed. *Continuity, coordination*, and *interpersonal elements of care* will also be part of quality measurement, although an approach to measuring these has not yet been devised. Characteristics of the health care *facility*, such as the privacy and dignity it affords patients and the cleanliness of the physical environment, will be considered. Finally, *staff morale and satisfaction* are viewed as integral to providing high-quality care and service and will be included in measurements of quality.

In addition to quantifying and reporting its performance using these indicators, HCHP will continue two existing quality assurance activities. The first is implicit review through medical record evaluation; trained record reviewers look at a sample of unusual deaths, readmissions within three days, and other "triggers." More such review is planned for the future. Second, the department will continue to respond to questions and concerns raised by clinical staff. For example, if a concern that the plan is not using a particular drug correctly arises, then the issue will be studied. As part of this problem-finding approach, the department director reads every complaint letter related to the delivery of care, reviews malpractice files, talks with department managers regularly, and "listens carefully at cocktail parties."

The plan is particularly concerned about telephone contact with members, believing that quality is at risk when improper information is provided or important questions go unasked. As a result, it has experimented with monitoring telephone conversations between clinical assistants and members to ensure accuracy and courtesy. Upon noting that the people answering the telephone after regular office hours were not familiar with basic diseases such as diabetes, a training program for clinical assistants was implemented. The program attempts to alert these staff to various symptoms and their possible implications and to their particular relevance when other conditions, such as diabetes, are present.

Another concern is Medicare beneficiaries' access to care. Under the new SeniorCare program, HCHP is monitoring Medicare members' access to initial appointments. The plan has established goals for seeing new Medicare members promptly and will measure its performance against them. HCHP hopes to see 35 percent of Medicare members within one month of their enrollment, 65 percent within two months, 80 percent within three months, and 95 percent within a year.

The automated medical records system is an asset to the quality measurement program. It has a series of automatic reminders to assist clinicians in monitoring particular conditions or risk factors. For example:

— Every abnormal Pap smear is flagged, and the computer prints a reminder to the physician that prompt follow-up is needed.

— Rubella-negative women who need immunization against German measles are identified.

— Every six months, physicians receive printouts of the patients in their panels who are taking diabetes medication; physicians thus know when these patients were last seen and when they last had a test for blood sugar.

— Patients taking lithium carbonate are identified so that dosages of the drug can be adjusted regularly.

— Reminders to vaccinate persons at high risk for influenza are printed periodically.

These reminders can also yield, when appropriate, statistics such as the percentage of members who should have received a flu vaccine but did not.

One traditional quality assurance activity is avoided by HCHP, namely, the routine examination of medical records for legibility, organization, and completeness. The vice president for quality measurement believes reviews of records are time-consuming, effect little change, and therefore provide small returns. HCHP conducts this type of review only to the extent required by state or federal authorities.

Relations With Hospitals

Relations with hospitals are colored strongly by HCHP's history. When HCHP first started operations, services were provided by physicians on the staff of two teaching hospitals of the Harvard Medical School: Brigham and Women's Hospital (known in Boston simply as "the Brigham") and Beth Israel Hospital. Even after HCHP hired its own medical staff, inpatient care continued to be provided predominately in these two hospitals—despite the fact that they are among the most expensive hospitals in the world. Discounted per diem rates were negotiated with these institutions.

As HCHP began to expand into the suburbs of Boston, it met intensifying competition from HMOs that used the less expensive community hospitals in those suburbs. HCHP would inevitably have to follow suit, and community hospital affiliations were established for some of its newest health centers.

In one community, resistance was encountered from the medical staff of the hospital with which HCHP wished to become affiliated. At about the same time, another hospital became available for affiliation. HCHP subsequently controlled the board, put it into operation as the HCHP Hopsital, and made it available to all the health centers. Although HCHP physicians are not required to use HCHP Hospital in preference to the Harvard teaching hospitals, the HCHP Hospital census stays reasonably close to its 69-bed capacity. The hospital is used for secondary care but also for some innovative purposes. When an HCHP member requires coronary bypass surgery, for example, the surgery is done in a Harvard teaching hospital, and the patient is cared for in that hospital for the first week after surgery. If further convalescence is required, the patient is moved to HCHP Hospital.

The entire relationship of HCHP to its affiliated hospitals may undergo a profound change because of an agreement in principle recently reached between the plan and the Brigham. Details have yet to be worked out, but the agreement essentially involves HCHP's contracting to use a specified, substantial number of Brigham beds each year at a deeply discounted rate. The number of beds involved increases by a specified amount in each of the next five years. The future of HCHP Hospital, and of the community hospitals with which some of the health centers are affiliated, has not been decided yet. Some HCHP executives think the HCHP Hospital will continue to operate as it does now; others think that it may be converted to some specialized use, such as rehabilitation. Under the expected terms of the agreement, however, HCHP Hospital will no longer have a strong price advantage over the Brigham.

Marketing and Member Relations

In describing marketing operations, HCHP marketing executives and staff tend to talk about three historical phases: the early years, when the principal competition was the Blue Cross-Blue Shield plan; the more recent years, in which competition from other HMOs has become steadily more intense; and the current phase, in which the marketing effort is being restructured in several ways.

In its first years, HCHP was the only HMO in the Boston area. As early as 1975, it had a significant price advantage over BC-BS, the primary competitor. Thus, HCHP marketing representatives spent relatively little time selling against competition. Rather, their principal task was to explain how HMOs work and how they differ from conventional health insurance plans. Marketing representatives were encouraged to prospect wherever they wished, and each representative developed his or her own "book of business." The approach was product-oriented. Sales presentations stressed the excellence of HCHP physicians and affiliated hospitals. The advantage of "everything in health care under one roof" was also emphasized, although marketing representatives were quick to point out that this concept is not for everyone.

Despite the rather low-key sales presentations, marketing overall was quite energetic. During this early stage of operations, HCHP was successful in signing up nearly 2,000 employer groups. Although federal qualification was useful in convincing employers of HCHP's legitimacy, the dual-choice mandate was rarely used; in fact, a large share of the 2,000 employer groups was signed up before HCHP became federally qualified. Since this early marketing push, HCHP has grown primarily by increasing membership in existing groups; today, the number of employers offering HCHP to their employees has grown only to about 2,200. In determining whether to enroll new employer groups (that is, the underwriting function), HCHP has been more liberal than many other HMOs. It has rarely turned down a group, for example, because of unfavorable demographics or expected high utilization.

After HCHP had been in operation a couple of years, other HMOs started to appear in the Boston area. Although competition increased, HCHP's marketing approach changed relatively little. Using the same sales appeal but adding HCHP's greater experience, HCHP increased enrollment within existing employer accounts. The plan decided to enroll Medicare beneficiaries. Its application to become a Medicare risk contract demonstration was being considered favorably when the Department of Health and Human Services decided not to contract for any more demonstrations. HCHP then decided to enroll Medicare beneficiaries under provisions of the Tax Equity and Fiscal Responsibility Act. It instituted a telemarketing campaign that quickly enrolled about 2,400 persons.

Within the last year, a major revamping of the HCHP marketing program has been initiated. Perhaps the most significant change is from a product-oriented to a market-oriented approach. Member surveys and other information on the market are being studied to determine how the plan can be made most attractive to members and prospective members. For example, a recent survey showed that members were not entirely happy with after-hours services; clinic schedules were modified to conform to member preferences more closely. New centers will be smaller, partially in response to expressed member preference.

The marketing staff has been reorganized into four groups, each focusing on a particular type of account: supergroups (very large employers, mostly government), existing accounts, small employers, and Medicare. HCHP had not pursued small employers previously.

Major components of the marketing program are being tailored to individual health centers. To compete more successfully in the suburbs, a separate premium structure for those areas has been introduced. More than a million dollars was budgeted for general advertising in 1985.

Organizationally, the marketing operations staff is divided into two levels. Account executives are responsible for enrolling new employer groups and for increasing enrollment in existing employer groups. Account service representatives are responsible for maintaining liaisons with and resolving problems for existing employer accounts. Representatives are recruited mainly from the HCHP health care delivery system, and their job is considered a stepping-stone to the account executive position, although account executives are also recruited from outside HCHP.

Training of marketing operations staff is done almost entirely on the job. After some initial orientation, new account executives accompany their experienced counterparts on actual sales calls. Training culminates in a sales presentation by the new account executive to the entire account executive group. Outside training courses have been used occasionally, but courses that are perceived as teaching highly aggressive selling are avoided. Account executives consider themselves to be educators rather than salespersons. They have been described as having more of a social service orientation than a sales orientation.

Compensation practices are consistent with this attitude. Until recently, account executives were paid base salaries only. A bonus program has now been introduced; under it, the entire marketing operations group shares in a modest bonus pool if enrollment goals are met. Bonuses based on individual performance are not used because they are thought to stimulate excessive internal competition. Although there has been considerable evolution in marketing operations, relatively little change has taken place in the member relations function. In most respects, the function is quite conventional; members' questions are answered and complaints investigated by experienced member relations representatives. Overall strengthening of this area is considered a high priority, even though HCHP's voluntary disenrollment rate is under 5 percent.

One unusual activity in this area is a survey of a random sample of members conducted every two months. Members are asked to rate the plan on some 20 different characteristics. Results are tabulated by health center, and the centers compete vigorously for the highest overall ratings.

Administration and Finance

Certainly a key factor in shaping HCHP's unique culture and performance has been the quality of its leadership. Another major determinant of the plan's sustained growth has been its ability to acquire sufficient capital to support its capital-intensive form of health care delivery. We discuss these two factors in the sections below, along with how HCHP's management information systems have evolved over the years.

Leadership

Primary responsibility for the leadership of HCHP is divided among three senior executives.

The president and chief executive officer, Thomas O. Pyle, is described as the visionary of the organization. He is said to have shaped the evolution of HCHP, including many of its innovations, since its early days. His attention is now directed mostly outward. In addition to his activities directly on behalf of HCHP itself, he is currently president of the Group Health Association of America and chairman of a malpractice insurance company. He is also chairman of the board of Managed Care, Inc., a new corporation set up by (but not owned by) HCHP to provide contract management to IPAs. He has been deeply involved in conceptualizing and negotiating the new contract with the Brigham.

Management of HCHP's two major operating components is divided between the medical director and chief operating officer, John M. Ludden, M.D., and the executive vice president and chief administrative officer, Richard J. Cannon. As described earlier, Ludden has complete line authority over the HCHP health care delivery system, and Cannon has identical authority over the "insurance" functions and certain other administrative functions of the plan.

Communications among the HCHP officers and senior executives are facilitated by three major committees: the policy group, the operations committee, and the benefits and contracts committee. It is through these committees that the two sides of the organization are linked together most effectively.

The policy group, chaired by the president, consists of the medical director, the executive vice president, and the chairman of the physicians council. It considers the broadest policy questions and approves all budgets; it meets on an ad hoc basis two to three times a month. A system of checks and balances is in place. The policy group has several lines of information besides the two senior officers described above: reporting directly to it are the vice president of quality measurement and the director of internal audit.

The operations committee considers significant operational issues every second week; it is chaired by the medical director. The benefits and contracts committee, headed by the executive vice president, meets monthly to consider additions to the benefits package, new services, and other modifications to HCHP's offerings. Most major decisions of the operations committee and the benefits and contracts committee are referred to the policy group for further action.

The board of directors of HCHP has 15 members. Among them are the president, the medical director, and two physicians elected by the physicians council. The other 11 members are primarily prominent business and professional people from the Boston area (although two are from outside the area).

This board recently replaced the former 28-member board, which is now known as the board of overseers.

The board of directors meets for at least three hours once a month. Its principal function is to review and approve proposals from the president and the policy group. The board sees its primary responsibility as strategic planning. This orientation is evident in its recent decision to appoint the Loran commission (named after the maritime navigational device). This commission, composed of prominent thinkers in the field of health care from the entire United States, is charged with creating a framework for dealing with the question of what new technologies HCHP should cover over the next decade. True to the academic tradition of

HCHP, the board anticipates that the work of the Loran commission will be of as much value to the entire HMO industry (or perhaps to the entire health care industry) as to HCHP itself.

HCHP is among the minority of HMOs that produce formal long-range plans. A vice president for planning, who reports to the executive vice president, is responsible for them. The planning function at HCHP may serve a slightly different purpose than it would in a proprietary organization. HCHP is a product-driven company rather than a market-driven one. That is, decisions are generally made not on the basis of market share or financial gain alone, but on the basis of these concerns in conjunction with the plan's medical values and patient care focus. In addition, the president is a highly intuitive leader whose style is complemented by a strategic plan that lays out steps and rationales for proposed decisions.

Three long-range plans have been prepared, one in 1976, one in 1983, and one in 1986.[5] They include an internal assessment of values, performance, strengths, and weaknesses; an analysis of the environment, including demographic trends and trends in the HMO and health care industry at large; opportunities for the future; and a conclusion with recommendations. As part of the plan, individual feasibility studies are done for each health center; these are updated yearly.

Two important goals of the new long-range plan have been enunciated: to grow at a rate of 15 to 20 percent a year, while controlling operations more tightly. Each of these goals is ambitious in itself; taken together, they are formidable, indeed.

While the planning process took one year in 1982–83, only six months were allocated to producing the 1986 plan, reflecting in part the need to adjust to a rapidly changing health care environment. The process is an iterative one, with ongoing feedback from the board and previews for senior management. The board's role is to make value decisions: it offers direction and will, for example, approve or disapprove ventures outside of HCHP's core business.

Much of the work of the board is done in committee, of which four are most important: finance, compensation, member services, and the physicians council. Each committee is chaired by a director and typically has one or two other directors as members, but most committees also have nondirectors as members.

Financial Management

The functions assigned to a chief financial officer in most organizations are divided between two officers in HCHP. The treasurer, who reports to the president, is responsible for raising and investing capital funds. He also monitors HCHP's premium structure, although he is not directly responsible for determining premiums. The vice president of financial operations, who reports to the executive vice president, is responsible for all other financial matters—principally accounting, budgeting, and operating systems (enrollment, underwriting, premium billing, rate setting, claims processing, and purchasing).

As a staff-model HMO, HCHP is capital-intensive. Reflecting a policy of borrowing up to capacity, HCHP's long-term debt ratio has been relatively stable. Until recently, the principal source of long-term funding has been tax-exempt revenue bonds issued through the Massachusetts Health and Educational Facilities Authority. The most recent borrowing through the authority was a $49,035,000 issue in December 1983. HCHP has nearly exhausted what it can get from this source and is turning to other organizations that can offer long-term funds on nearly as attractive a basis. A new five-year plan to raise an additional $25 million has been developed. Funds derived from long-term debt are augmented by setting aside 2.5 percent above depreciation for capital investment.

With respect to operating expenses, HCHP has not been concerned until quite recently about being a high-cost producer. This was particularly true in its earliest years. One executive described this period by saying, "The plan's early founders loaded an incredible amount of innovative baggage on a fragile organization—five to ten variations on the Kaiser model." Experimentation was going on concurrently, for example, in the areas of medical records, nursing roles, and benefit packages. There were many relationships to manage, and the organization was a patchwork quilt of subcontracts.

The prevailing wisdom has been that HCHP can compete successfully in the marketplace with premiums 5 percent above those of its strongest competitors. Therefore, there was little emphasis on budgetary control during HCHP's formative years. This relaxed attitude was reinforced by relatively stable profit margins through the 1970s, despite rapid expansion of the plan and continued experimentation in the health care delivery system.

This complacency was shattered by the financial setback of 1981, described earlier, which revealed shortcomings in HCHP's management controls, particularly in its management information systems. (Responses to these deficiencies are discussed in the next section.)

As HCHP moved to correct these problems, the urgency of the task was underscored by rapid intensification of price competition after 1982, both from other HMOs and from BC-BS. The most visible reactions have been a sudden emphasis, in 1985, on budgetary controls and a close scrutiny of every element of cost throughout the plan. A five-pronged strategy for containing or lowering costs has been developed:

— Buy inpatient services cheaper

— Increase physician productivity

— Increase standardization across health centers

— Put more compensation at risk

— Modify HCHP's high-style approach

This new emphasis on controlling costs, incidentally, may be the first tangible demonstration of the value of the HCHP commitment to physician managers. The costs on which the greatest constraints focus are, of course, costs related to direct provision of patient care. In most HMOs, this would immediately pit physicians against nonphysician managers. At HCHP, however, the individuals doing the most severe cost cutting are the physician managers themselves, so a we-they dichotomy is less likely to emerge.

One group of costs being scrutinized with particular care is outside medical services. These are increasing at 15 to 25 percent annually. A concerted effort is being made to bring some of these services in-house, and preferred provider arrangements are being considered for others. Another area in which a sharp reaction to price competition can be seen readily is the HCHP rate structure. In the past, HCHP adhered closely to a simple, two-tiered structure, even though this often made it difficult to sell the plan to young married couples. ("Why should we, as a couple, pay more than twice as much for coverage as a single person?") Furthermore, the plan adhered closely to a single, community-rated premium structure for its entire service area, even though this made it difficult for HCHP to compete in the suburbs against HMOs that use less expensive community hospitals.

Although HCHP continues to be relatively conservative in its approach to rate setting, it has departed from its insistence on a single, two-tiered structure. It is moving cautiously into three-tiered rates where necessary in order to compete effectively with other insurers, and it has recently received federal approval of a separate, lower rate structure for certain Boston suburban areas. The possibility of offering high- and low-cost benefit options is being explored. The increasing complexity of rate setting at HCHP has prompted the director of operating systems (who has direct responsibility for rate setting) to develop a rate-setting model on a microcomputer; he says that he no longer can do without such a model.

Underlying this shift is a more subtle shift from budget-driven rate setting to market-driven rate setting. Until the last year or two, rates were determined by projecting the costs of providing the type of care HCHP considers to be consistent with its image. If this resulted in a relatively substantial year-to-year increase in rates, that was considered an inherent cost of doing things the HCHP way. Competitive discomfort was eased by the fact that health care costs in Boston were rising faster than in the nation as a whole. Now, however, rate setting begins with a statement such as, "The premium this year cannot increase more than 5 percent," and costs are expected to be pared until that result is achieved.

Management Information Systems

Management of HCHP recognizes that the plan has been underinvested in core administrative systems throughout most of its history. This has come about for two reasons. The first was the relatively relaxed attitude toward budgetary controls until the last year or two, as described above. The second has been HCHP's preoccupation with the COSTAR (Computer-Stored Ambulatory Record) system, a pioneering venture in automating medical records. COSTAR is recognized nationally as probably the most sophisticated approach yet developed to computer-assisted storage and retrieval of medical records information. At one point, it was seen as having potential value for administrative purposes, but this potential has never been realized. Against this background, HCHP developed its core administrative systems in a rather disjointed way.

The *enrollment* system was developed as an adjunct to the COSTAR system on in-house Digital Equipment Corporation (DEC 1170) hardware (hardware that is now totally obsolete). The MUMPS (Massachusetts General Hospital Utility Multi-Programming System) software used with this system, however, is not geared toward large-scale data manipulation, so it was nearly impossible to realize most of the administrative potential of the enrollment files. In 1983, the enrollment system was separated from the COSTAR system and placed on new, in-house Hewlett-Packard (HP 3000) hardware.

Until 1976, *premium billing* was done for HCHP by BC-BS. When formal relations with BC-BS were severed in 1976, the premium billing function was moved to a service bureau. In 1986, HCHP will convert to an in-house system.

Although the *claims processing* function is supported in some incidental ways by computers, it is still essentially a manual system—even though the volume of claims being processed will reach 160,000 next year. Each claim is checked manually against medical records and the enrollment files. It is then adjudicated by a claims processor, after which it is checked manually for coordination of benefits. Until recently, the disposition of each claim was recorded on a 5" by 8" card; this part of the process has now been replaced by a computerized claims logging system.

Purchasing and receiving are entirely manual processes.

As noted earlier, some of the deficiencies of this situation became painfully evident in 1981. A major systems development effort was started in 1982. This effort is expected to be completed by the end of 1986, by which time the total investment in it is expected to reach $2.5 million. As part of the effort,

— All systems will be brought in-house.

— Important systems that are now manual—principally claims processing and purchasing-receiving—will be automated.

— Major systems will eventually be integrated on HP 3000 hardware, which will replace the DEC 1170 hardware.

— A database management approach will be incorporated into the integrated systems, and increased emphasis will be placed on database security.

— The COSTAR system will be moved from the DEC 1170 hardware to later generation equipment, a major undertaking. This will commence with a pilot plan in one health center.

— The use of personal computers will be encouraged throughout HCHP. The possibility of equipping marketing representatives with portable terminals that can tap into the HP 3000 mainframe will be considered seriously.

— More attention will be given to technological planning to avoid the current practice of playing catch-up.

Teaching and Research

A commitment to teaching and research is part of what makes HCHP unique, and ongoing support of these activities is seen as a critical, shared value. Teaching and research programs are funded through a combination of premium revenues and grants from external sources. Currently, 1 percent of the plan's premium revenues is earmarked for these programs.

The HCHP Teaching Center

The mission of HCHP's Teaching Center is to establish a place for HMOs in the training of health care professionals. The center is designed to teach physicians and other clinicians-in-training the skills, attitudes, and knowledge they will need to practice in the future, particularly those attributes needed to practice within prepaid health care systems. The center is committed to developing new methods of training clinicians while ensuring feedback into the management and practice of medicine at HCHP.

These are four main areas of education and training:

— Medicine: projects include the development of a model primary care residency and primary care electives, and the teaching of the introduction to clinical medicine course to Harvard Medical School students.

— Nursing: the focus is on an expanded role for nurse practitioners in collaborative practice with physicians. Nurse practitioner students are given an opportunity to be part of a clinical team; specialty training programs in areas such as geriatrics, home care, and women's health are under development.

— Management: HCHP sponsors two management fellows each year and hires about six to eight management interns each summer.

— Mental health: The plan has a one-year program to teach cost-constrained shorter-term therapy to advanced mental health clinicians (psychiatry residents in their final year of training, postdoctoral psychologists, and postmaster's degree clinicians with two to three years' experience).

There are also faculty development and other teaching programs, many of which are efforts to improve communication between clinicians and patients.

The Institute For Health Research

The Institute for Health Research is a joint venture with Harvard University that began in July 1983. The institute is an independent research arm that uses HCHP as a laboratory and a resource. Its work in health policy and health services research, however, is independent of the plan's agenda.

The major areas of research in which the institute is now engaged are the following:

— Mental Health: The institute has a diversified research agenda that specializes in methodology, prevention, behavioral determinants of utilization, and clinical trials.

— Assessment of health practices: This area includes studies in technology assessment and clinical decision making, with an emphasis on using clinical investigators both inside and outside the institute.

— Indexes of system performance: This new area of research will complement the efforts of HCHP's quality of care measurement program described above. The purpose is to develop rigorous and credible methods of comparing systems of care in terms of outcomes.

Notes

1. Gordon T. Moore, "History of the Harvard Community Health Plan," in *Health Maintenance Organizations and Academic Medical Centers*, eds. James I. Hudson and Madeline M. Nevins (Menlo Park, N.J.: Henry J. Kaiser Family Foundation, 1981), pp. 190–209.
2. See Elena T. Blakeley, "Benefits Coverage versus Premium Level, an

Ethical Tradeoff: Harvard Community Health Plan's Experience," paper presented at the Group Health Institute, Philadelphia, June 1984.

3. A new HCHP urgent care center is under construction at the Brigham and Women's Hospital, adjacent to that hospital's own emergency department.

4. The policy group, composed of the president, the medical director, the executive vice president, and the chairperson of the physicians council, considers broad policy questions and approves all budgets. It is discussed in more detail later in this chapter.

5. The plan was not finished at the time this study was done.

23

Success Factors

All the strengths described in chapter 22 contributed in some way to HCHP's success, but three factors seem to have special significance.

Sense of Identity and Direction

The plan has an exceptional sense of identity and direction. In discussions with people throughout HCHP's management ranks, it quickly becomes evident that they know what HCHP stands for and where it is going. This attitude is so pervasive that it is difficult to capture it well on paper, but at least three elements convey some sense of how it dominates the way HCHP management behaves.

First, reflecting its Harvard Medical School origin, HCHP is dedicated to innovating health care delivery concepts in the HMO setting. Comments were made in several of our interviews suggesting that HCHP sees itself not only as a provider of high-quality medical care, but also as a pathfinder in the HMO industry.

This can be seen in HCHP's typical approach to developing new systems and techniques. It often opts for concepts that have potential value for the entire industry, not just for HCHP, even though this may add substantial cost. A conspicuous example is the COSTAR medical information system, which is far more sophisticated than the systems most HMOs use but is a true and significant innovation in this area. One purpose of HCHP's venture into the IPA field, in the form of its managed care affiliate, was described as seizing an opportunity to learn and perhaps to provide leadership in this different approach to providing prepaid health care. This tendency to experiment reinforces the academic tradition that has been part of the HCHP culture since the organization's inception.

A predilection for innovation might lead to disaster without some way to channel it. At HCHP, this is found in strategic planning, toward which both the CEO and the board direct much of their energy.

Thomas Pyle, the CEO, generally spurs the strategic planning effort. Pyle is regarded within HCHP and throughout much of the HMO industry as an imaginative thinker, possibly a visionary. The board's role in strategic planning involves more than merely acting as a sounding board for the CEO. It has vigorous discussions about planning issues and does not always endorse management proposals. Board members interact directly with the vice president of planning and other senior staff members with respect to various aspects of HCHP's long-range plan.

One of the most visible demonstrations of the importance HCHP attaches to strategic planning is the CEO's initiation of the Loran commission, described earlier. Characteristically, the chairman of the board commented that this commission may provide some valuable direction to the entire HMO industry.

Finally, a conspicuous product of this sense of identity and direction is an exceptional esprit de corps in the organization, particularly at the senior levels. Managers are convinced that they are building and managing a unique health care enterprise and that their colleagues in this enterprise are simply the best in the business. Their enthusiasm leads them to pour in far more personal energy than the minimum demands of their jobs.

Clinical Excellence

HCHP has been quite successful in communicating to the public, to its members and their employers, and to its own staff an image of uncompromising clinical performance. At least four strategies have been orchestrated skillfully to accomplish this.

First is the unquestionable distinction HCHP derives from its use of the Harvard name. Even though there is no formal tie between HCHP and Harvard Medical School, HCHP plays up its continuing association with the school. A significant percentage of its medical staff are graduates of Harvard Medical School or have completed residencies in the school's teaching hospitals.

It must be noted that the Harvard name has not been an unmixed blessing. It has attracted resentment from some quarters, particularly from competitors, who see it as an unfair advantage. Furthermore, the Harvard name has more luster outside Boston than it does in some parts of Boston, especially in several low-income areas, so it is less of a universal marketing asset than might be assumed. There are more than a few people who hoped in the early days that HCHP would fail, to teach "the Harvard crowd" a lesson.

A second important strategy is that of using teaching hospitals affiliated with Harvard Medical School for most hospitalizations. This practice and its corollary, that most HCHP physicians have admitting privileges at at least one of the Harvard teaching hospitals, are seen by many people as convincing evidence of clinical excellence.

A third potent strategy contributing to the image of clinical excellence is HCHP's commitment to the concept of the physician manager. The people that both staff and members see as being in charge are almost always physicians. The policy that physician managers must continue to see patients ensures that they do not lose this visibility. Although other HMOs place physicians in management roles, few, if any, others are as committed to doing so in most key management slots at every level of the organization.

A fourth and somewhat derivative strategy is HCHP's highly selective physician recruitment program. The combination of the association with Harvard Medical School, the academic ambiance, the reputation for clinical excellence, and the emphasis on physician managers makes HCHP extraordinarily attractive to many physicians with impeccable credentials.

Effective Marketing of Clinical Excellence

Although clinical excellence clearly implies high-quality care, it is equally valuable as a marketing tool. HCHP has been successful in translating clinical excellence into sustained membership growth, mostly by emphasizing the theme of clinical excellence subtly but effectively in its entire spectrum of marketing messages.

The theme is communicated most directly in marketing representatives' presentations to employers and prospective members. Both the practice of using Harvard teaching hospitals and the strength of the medical staff are featured in these presentations. Access to a wide variety of board-certified specialists under one roof is a collateral message.

These messages are reinforced, often obliquely, in HCHP advertising. One example is the mileage HCHP derived from publicizing its first member to receive a heart transplant. This not only reassured members about the comprehensiveness of HCHP's services, but it also conveyed the message that HCHP stays right at medicine's leading edge. Even more subtle themes are projected by HCHP's dedication to excellent style in its printed materials and advertising campaigns. Consistent attention to these details conveys the message that HCHP is a "class act."

Marketing success is not, of course, built solely on effective image building. The fact that HCHP was the first significant HMO in the Boston market cannot be discounted. Being first allowed it to concentrate initially on rapid membership growth from broad coverage of an essentially uncontested market, thus achieving break-even status early in its history. Only later did the plan undertake the more difficult marketing task of attaining greater penetration within existing accounts. This approach has worked well; as noted earlier, membership has grown vigorously in every year of HCHP's history.

Appendix

Overview of Previous Research

$\mathbf{A}$ lot has been written about HMO success and performance. The literature includes general work on excellence or success in business, excellence in health care organizations (Shortell 1985), the performance of HMOs in terms of utilization and cost control (Luft 1981), attempts to differentiate between successful and unsuccessful HMOs (Wasserman 1976, U.S. General Accounting Office 1978, Jurgovan & Blair, Inc. 1979), and various case studies of particular HMOs. These case studies focus on indicators of financial performance (Touche Ross & Company 1982, 1983) and documentation of HMO failures (American Association of Foundations for Medical Care 1981), successes (American Association of Foundations for Medical Care 1980), and turnarounds (Staff of Physicians Health Plan 1980).

We address here primarily success factors that are internal to the organization, although selected studies of external factors such as market demographics and the nature of the competition are also reported. Moreover, we restrict ourselves largely to discussion of factors that various authors postulate are related to HMO success or failure. Thus, works dealing with general management and case studies of individual HMOs are not reviewed.

Internal Factors for Success

In a comprehensive review of the literature through 1981, Luft and Trauner (1981) synthesized the descriptive studies on factors affecting HMO performance. They grouped the studies into six in-

ternal management categories, plus the external environment.
The following are their major findings from the literature:

— *Sponsorship and goals.* These reflect the attitudes and
orientation of the professional staff. Lack of sufficient
commitment to the HMO principle has been cited as a
cause of failure in some IPAs. Consumer involvement
and for-profit or nonprofit status appear to have no consistent effect.

— *Organizational and administrative structure.* Low administrative costs in relation to revenues may be more important than overall growth in enrollment. There is great
variation in the time required to break even and in enrollment size at that point. IPAs are less costly to develop
than group or staff models. Inadequate managerial experience has consistently been related to failure. Ultimate
success is contingent upon establishing effective control
over utilization.

— *Methods of paying physicians.* Risk-sharing agreements
whereby physicians share in the HMO's financial gains
and losses can improve performance. HMOs may be adversely affected when physicians in the plan continue to
treat fee-for-service patients: such physicians may shift
costs from their own patients to the HMO and may be
less responsive to HMO patients.

— *Physician staffing.* An HMO's success is directly related
to its ability to recruit a cadre of physicians who are committed to practicing cost-conscious medicine. HMOs that
start operations with a full range of specialists and too
few primary care physicians are at a competitive disadvantage. Sudden, unexpected growth in enrollment can
create significant staffing difficulties.

— *Control of hospital services.* The HMO that controls its
own hospital saves physician and consultant time, avoids
duplicating equipment and personnel, and exerts more
control over admissions, discharges, and bed allocation.
Filling a hospital, however, requires a large enrollment in
a densely populated area. The alternative is to contract
with hospitals and negotiate rates. An HMO's best opportunity for negotiating discounts may be with hospitals
that have excess bed capacity. On the other hand, the
HMO may choose to forego the discount and use a facility

with a high occupancy rate in which pressure for space has created efficient patterns of utilization.

— *Marketing of services.* Six components of a successful HMO marketing program are (1) evaluation of enrollment prospects in specific groups, (2) determination of appropriate premiums and benefit packages based upon knowledge of the competitive environment, (3) development of presentations for key health benefits personnel and union officials, (4) production of marketing materials, (5) servicing of existing accounts, and (6) knowledge of the competitive environment. HMOs need a clear marketing strategy that is understood and accepted by management and the medical staff. Overselling may lead to unrealistic expectations by members, and that can hamper efficient use of the HMO's staff and facilities.

Strumpf and Garramone (1976) found two internal factors contributing to success: *a nucleus of committed physicians* and *sufficient start-up capital.* They cite three reasons for failure: lack of commitment on the part of the sponsoring organization, lack of appropriate management structure or expertise, and overly optimistic projections of market share, usually resulting from ignorance of barriers to acceptance by consumers and providers.

Wasserman (1976) studied 6 successful plans and 12 failures. Factors correlating with success included *a lower ratio of administrative staff to enrollees, incentives to control hospital utilization,* and *organizational balance,* a quality Wasserman defines as the ability to integrate functions and to understand the implications of management decisions for all parts of the organization. Attributes of failed HMOs were higher administrative expenses, more emphasis on the profit motive and greater use of proprietary hospitals, less emphasis on quality, less group orientation among physician staff, fewer incentives for controlling hospital use, and greater dependence on state Medicaid contracts.

The General Accounting Office (1978) evaluated 14 federally qualified HMOs to see if they complied with the requirements of the 1973 HMO Act. The findings showed most plans in compliance, although GAO expressed concern about the ability of some of the HMOs to achieve financial independence within five years. Specifically, GAO was pessimistic about the long-term financial independence of six plans and concerned about another three. It concluded that *HMOs depending heavily on health care resources in the fee-for-service sector lack control over a significant portion of their costs* (although utilization is controlled, the decision making of managers is not). Second, *an HMO's pricing strategy is as important as cost control* (underpricing services to be competitive can cause long-term problems). Third, *effective management is critical for HMO success.*

Jurgovan & Blair, Inc. (1979) studied data submitted to the federal government by 40 qualified HMOs. Their purpose was to identify and rank factors that both characterize successful HMOs and discriminate between successful and struggling or failed plans. They tracked four categories of expense as a percentage of revenue (total, administrative, medical, and hospital); hospital statistics (patient-days per thousand members, discharge rate, average length of stay); and deficit per member per month. They found that *low administrative expense as a percentage of revenue was the variable most highly correlated with HMO success.*

Touche Ross & Co. (1982, 1983) describe trends in the HMO industry for potential investors. Their studies highlight four key elements of successful HMOs: *market acceptance* (noted as the most important factor), *effective relationships with physicians, established cost controls, and capable board and top management.* The studies also provide information on the financial characteristics of HMOs, including their capital needs. They profile three HMOs, two of which are included in our study—Maxicare and U.S. Healthcare (HMO-PA).

Harrison and Kimberly (1982) state that "HMOs don't have to fail," although the difficulties of managing physicians, instituting fiscal controls and appropriate management information systems, and managing growth and change have resulted in HMO failures. Three common deficiencies cited by the authors are lack of management skills, lack of understanding of the HMO environment, and lack of ability to manage change.

External Factors for Success

The role of external factors has been addressed in case studies of market areas (typically, metropolitan) and of individual HMOs, as well as in econometric (statistical) analyses. Luft and Trauner in their review (1981) found evidence to support the role of certain external factors in promoting or impeding HMO development. They reported that:

— Local medical community resistance can slow HMO growth.

— Restrictive state laws appear no longer to impair HMO development, although federal requirements for a broad benefit package and community rating may place some plans at a competitive disadvantage.

— HMOs seem to have developed first in areas characterized by a large, dense, and growing population, especially when that population was relatively affluent, unionized, liberal, and covered by health insurance.

— The local health insurance market, particularly community norms for the number of health plan options offered and the level of employer or union contribution, can have a major impact on HMOs.

Various regression analyses have also been performed. Goldberg and Greenberg (1981) found HMO growth to be enhanced by high and rapidly growing hospital costs, highly mobile populations, and a high percentage of physicians in group practice. Another study found HMO enrollment to be negatively related to the percentage of physicians between the ages of 45 and 64 and positively related to per capita income (Morrisey and Ashby 1982). It also found market share to be negatively related to the percentage of the population under age 14, the percentage over age 65, the percentage female, and the percentage nonwhite.

As part of a review performed by Lewin and Associates, Over, Watt, and Roenigk (1983) identified the following variables as favorably affecting HMO growth:

— Favorable business and physician attitudes

— A high-growth area with mobile, especially young, populations without strong ties to particular physicians

— Large employers with well-paid employees

— Little unionization

— High medical costs as well as high ratios of physicians and beds to population

Building upon earlier research, Over, Watt, and Roenigk modeled group and staff versus IPA enrollment and found the following:

— IPAs were commonly formed as a competitive response to group- or staff-model HMOs.

— HMOs tended to form in areas of high population density (IPA market share, as opposed to likelihood of formation, tended to be lower in high-density areas than did group and staff market shares) and, although HMOs tended to form in areas with higher numbers of recent immigrants, their market share, unexpectedly, was lower in those areas.

— Physician and hospital supply affected IPA but not group or staff market share.

References

American Association of Foundations for Medical Care. 1980. *Physicians Association of Clackamas County; CompreCare; United Healthcare.* Washington, D.C.: Government Printing Office.

———. 1981. *ChoiceCare Health Services.* Washington, D.C.: Government Printing Office.

Goldberg, Lawrence G., and Warren Greenberg. 1981. "Determinants of HMO Enrollment and Growth." *Health Services Research* 16: 421–38.

Harrison, Deborah, and John Kimberly. 1982. "HMOs Don't Have to Fail." *Harvard Business Review* 60 (July-August): 115–24.

Jurgovan & Blair, Inc. 1979. *Health Maintenance Organization Viability.* Rockville, Md.: JBI.

Luft, Harold S. 1981. *Health Maintenance Organizations: Dimensions of Performance.* New York: John Wiley & Sons.

Luft, Harold S., and Joan B. Trauner. 1981. *The Operations and Performance of Health Maintenance Organizations: A Synthesis of Findings From Health Service Research.* San Francisco: Institute for Health Policy Studies.

Morrisey, Michael W., and Cynthia S. Ashby. 1982. "An Empirical Analysis of HMO Market Share." *Inquiry* 19 (Summer): 136–49.

Over, A. Mead, Jr., J. Michael Watt, and Dale Roenigk. 1983. *Private Sector Health Care Initiatives: Market Area Characteristics Analysis.* Prepared for the Office of the Assistant Secretary for Planning and Evaluation, DHHS, contract no. HHS-100-82-0031. Washington, D.C.: Lewin and Associates, Inc.

Shortell, Stephen M. 1985. "High-Performing Healthcare Organizations: Guidelines for the Pursuit of Excellence." *Hospital & Health Services Administration* 30 (July-August): 7–35.

Staff of Physicians Health Plan. 1980. "The Physicians Health Plan of Minnesota: A Case Study of Utilization Controls in an IPA." Unpublished paper supported by the Office of Health Maintenance Organizations.

Strumpf, George B., and Marie A. Garramone. 1976. "Why Some HMOs Develop Slowly." *Public Health Reports* 91 (November-December): 496–503.

Touche Ross & Co. 1982. *Investor's Guide to Health Maintenance Organizations.* Washington, D.C.: Government Printing Office.

————. 1983. *The 1983 Investor's Guide to Health Maintenance Organizations.* Washington, D.C.: Government Printing Office.

U.S. General Accounting Office. 1978. *Can Health Maintenance Organizations Be Successful? An Analysis of 14 Federally Qualified HMOs.* Washington, D.C.: GAO.

Wasserman, Fred W. 1976. "Health Maintenance Organizations: Determinants of Failure or Success." Doctoral dissertation, University of California, Los Angeles.

About the Authors

PETER D. FOX is a vice president of Lewin and Associates, a Washington-based research and consulting firm, where he has worked on a variety of topics in the areas of health financing and alternative delivery systems. His clients have been both public agencies and private organizations, including the U.S. Department of Health and Human Services, HMOs, insurance carriers, various provider groups interested in alternative delivery systems, health care coalitions, private foundations and associations, pharmaceutical and medical device companies, and state and local governments. For 11 years before joining the firm in 1981, Dr. Fox served in a variety of positions in the federal government, the latest of which was director of the Office of Policy Analysis in the Health Care Financing Administration. He has also worked for Stanford Research Institute (now called SRI International) and the Stanford University School of Medicine. Dr. Fox has published articles on such topics as alternative delivery systems, physician reimbursement, physician utilization patterns, mental health program evaluation, and long-term care. He also wrote, with Willis B. Goldbeck and Jacob J. Spies, *Health Care Cost Management: Private Sector Initiatives*, which was published in 1984 by Health Administration Press. He has a Ph.D. in business administration from Stanford University, an M.S. in management from the Massachusetts Institute of Technology, and an A.B. from Haverford College.

LUANN HEINEN is a consultant at Lewin and Associates in Washington, D.C., where she specializes in health care financing issues. She has worked on projects for insurance carriers, HMOs, university medical centers, pharmaceutical and medical products companies, and the federal government. Before that, she worked at Duke University's Center for Health Policy Research and Education and at Urban Systems Research and Engineering in Cambridge, Mass. Ms. Heinen has a master's of public policy from the Kennedy School of Government at Harvard University and an A.B. in human biology from Stanford University.

RICHARD J. STEELE is vice president of Birch & Davis Associates, Inc., of Silver Spring, Maryland. He has been a professional management consultant for 37 years, most recently focused exclusively on the health care industry. He collaborated with LuAnn Heinen on the Harvard Community Health Plan study and directed three of the other case studies described in this book.